REFLEXOLOGY
A PRACTICAL GUIDE

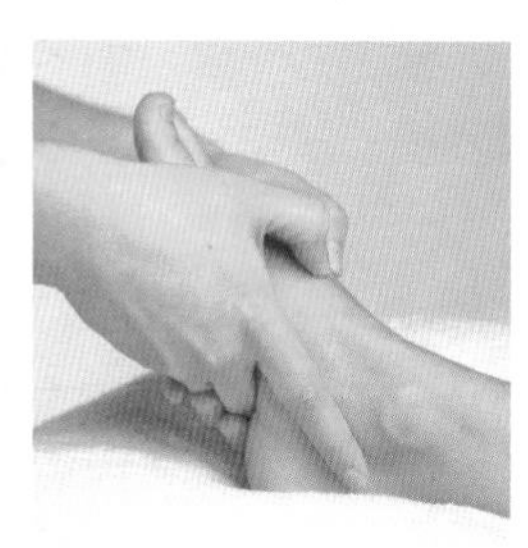
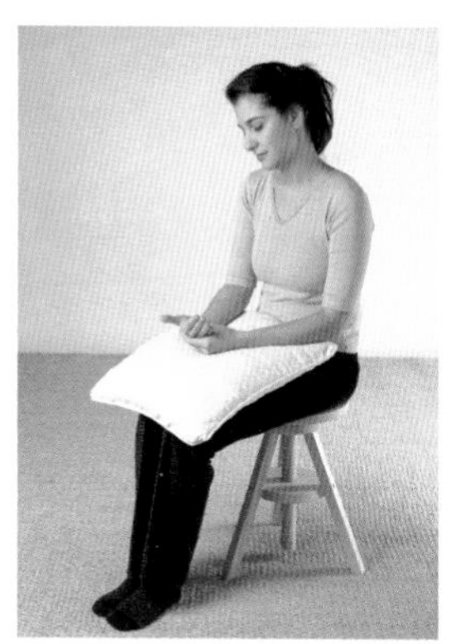
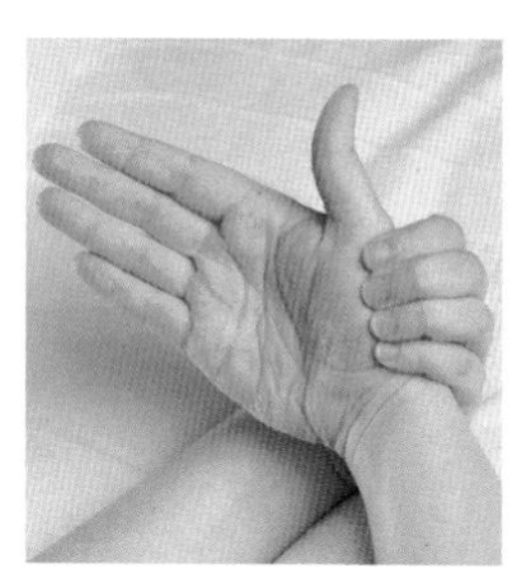

JOANNA TREVELYAN

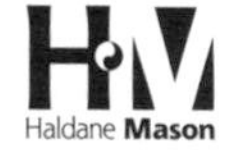

First published in the UK in 2001 by
Haldane Mason Ltd
59 Chepstow Road
London W2 5BP
email: haldane.mason@dial.pipex.com

ISBN: 1-902463-48-X

A HALDANE MASON BOOK

Editors: Ambreen Husain, Elizabeth Rowe
Designer: Rachel Clark
Consultants: Simon Duncan, Helen Venn-Brown MBChA MSSCh MAR
Models: Helen Venn-Brown, Cristiane Guida de Camargo

Colour reproduction by CK Litho Ltd, UK
Printed in China

Picture Acknowledgements
All photographs by Sue Ford, with the exception of the following:
Werner Forman Archive 4. The photograph on page 7 is reproduced by courtesy of The International School of Reflexology & Meridian Therapy.

Important

The information in this book is generally applicable but is not tailored to specific circumstances or individuals. The author and publishers can accept no responsibility for any problems arising from following the information given in this book. Safety information is supplied which should be read before attempting any of the treatments. If in doubt about any of the techniques described, please consult your doctor or reflexology practitioner.

Contents

Introduction

Most of us have experienced the pleasure of massaging our tired feet after a strenuous walk, or the relief of being able to put our feet up at the end of a long day. Taking care of our feet seems to make our entire body feel good, so a therapy that works on this part of the body (and occasionally on the hands too) to improve the health and sense of well-being of the whole person is one which appeals to many.

Historical background

We can be fairly sure that the therapeutic use of hand and foot pressure for the treatment of pain, as well as for various other ailments, was being used in China and India more than 5,000 years ago. A stone relief and paintings found in the Physician's Tomb at Saqqara in Egypt suggest that the Ancient Egyptians were also using some form of therapeutic manipulation of the feet and hands around 2500–2300 BC. Moreover, there is a long tradition of foot massage among some native American tribes, who believe that our feet are our connection with the Earth, although we do not know when this practice started. The reflexology described in this book, however, has more recent origins.

In the early 20th century, an American ear, nose and throat specialist called William H. Fitzgerald (1872–1942) published reports of his discovery, albeit accidental, that gentle pressure applied to specific parts of the hand or foot caused partial anaesthesia in areas of the ear, nose and throat. He claimed that, by using pressure points on the hands and feet, he was able to perform minor surgery without using an anaesthetic. Fitzgerald tried to map these areas or 'zones'. In 1917, he published a joint paper with a Dr Edwin Bowers which described 'reflex zone therapy'. This identified 10 zones running through the body and included 'maps' of the internal organs reflected on the hands and feet. Controlled pressure with the fingers and thumbs at the ends of these 'zones' was said to produce a response elsewhere in the body. 'Reflexology', claimed Fitzgerald and Bowers, could have an effect – which could be beneficial – on individual organs and the inter-relationship between organs and other body systems.

Since then, other people have developed the principles and practice of reflexology further. Among them was Dr Joseph Riley who, in 1920, described the horizontal zones of the feet. Then Eunice D. Ingham, a research assistant of Riley's, attempted to define the precise zone pathways. She argued that all parts of the body could be affected by pressure on clearly defined areas of the feet – particularly the soles. The treatment techniques she developed became known as the 'Ingham Reflex Method of Compression Massage'.

In the 1960s, a student of Ingham's called Doreen Bailey introduced reflexology to the UK and opened up a training school for therapists. Over the past 40 years, the popularity of reflexology has been increasing steadily. Today it is acknowledged to be one of the most popular complementary therapies.

This stone relief from the tomb of two priests overseeing royal manicurists in Egypt depicts a foot massage and, possibly, a hand massage or manicure.

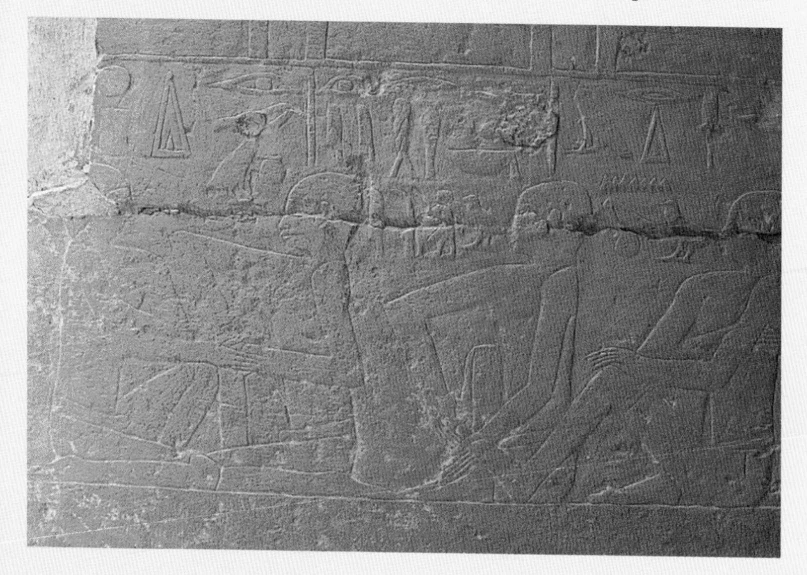

What *is* *Reflexology?*

Reflexology involves the application of varying degrees of pressure to one part of the body – usually the feet (and occasionally the hands) – in order to produce beneficial effects in other parts of the body. A number of different techniques have developed, but they are all based on the premise that treating the foot can have a healing effect on the whole body.

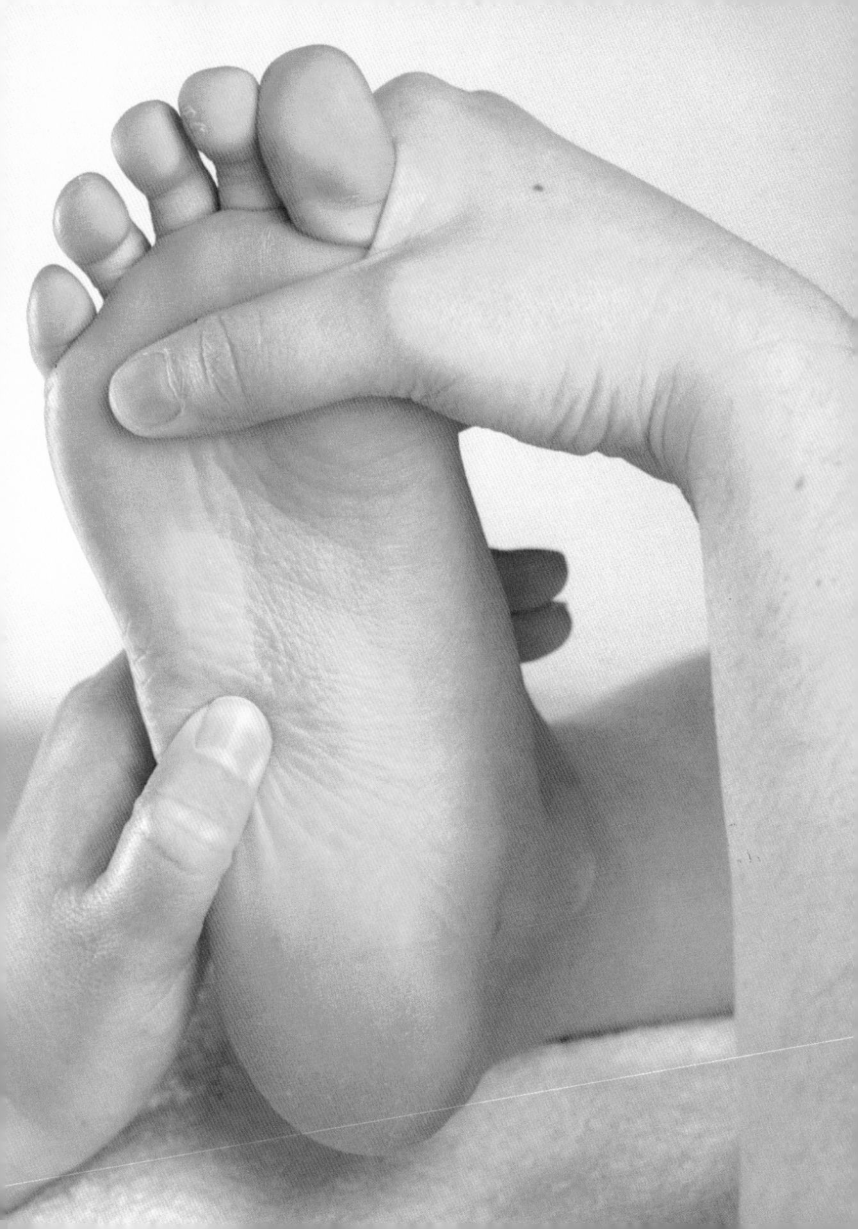

Reflexology today

Over the years, various techniques based on traditional reflexology have been developed, with some more popular than others. Although scientific research into this therapy remains minimal, it is used widely in health care, and is seen as an effective all-round therapy.

The Metamorphic Technique

This approach was devised in the 1960s by the British naturopath and reflexologist Robert St John, who originally called it 'prenatal therapy'. Proponents argue that it is neither a therapy nor strictly a treatment, but instead practitioners act as catalysts, enabling patients to heal themselves.

The basis of the Metamorphic Technique is the belief that ill-health can often be traced back to problems before birth. St John came to believe not only that every part of the body is represented on the foot, but also that the time spent in the womb is mapped out on the side of the foot, along points known as spinal reflexes. Mental, physical, emotional and spiritual patterns set before birth can, he said, be felt in the altered states of the foot's surfaces.

With a light, feathery touch, practitioners of this technique seek to help the individual release any energy blockages, and so alter the states that led to ill-health or stress. No one knows how this technique works, but its practitioners claim great success, particularly with people who feel they are in a rut, who are suffering from anxiety or who want to change in some way. It has also been used to help with a variety of conditions, such as cancer, multiple sclerosis and ME.

Vacuflex reflexology

This system was devised during the 1970s by Inge Dougans, a Danish reflexologist. Dougans believed that reflexology works by treating the meridians described in Chinese medicine, along which 'chi' energy flows. Vacuflex reflexology provides a way of stimulating all the reflex areas at the same time at the beginning of a treatment session.

Special Vacuflex 'boots' are worn for the first stage of a treatment. These are made of felt and are fitted around the feet. The air inside is then withdrawn by a vacuum pump, squeezing the feet firmly and thus stimulating all the reflexes at once.

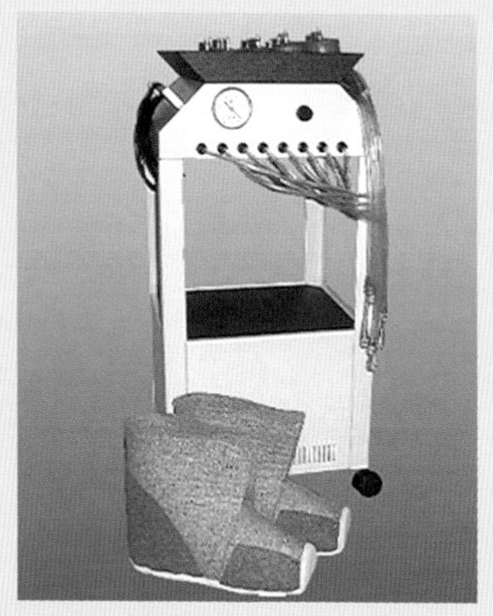

After the Vacuflex boots are fitted round the patient's feet, the air is withdrawn by a vacuum pump.

Stimulating the reflex points results in the corresponding areas of the body being stimulated. After about five minutes, the boots are removed and the therapist quickly looks for areas of discoloration on the feet. These marks, which are said to indicate areas of congestion and ill-health in the body, usually disappear after 20–30 seconds. Over several sessions, progress is measured by the change in size of the area of discoloration at each successive session.

For the second stage of treatment, the therapist places silicon pads of different sizes and combinations on specific reflex points which lie along energy meridians on the feet, legs, hands and arms. The pads are held in place by gentle suction, and are said to stimulate the meridians. After a few seconds, the pads are removed. Therapists claim that this system is an effective way to treat a wide range of conditions.

Research

Many therapists have written about their successful use of reflexology, and patients too have shared their success stories with newspaper and magazine readers. Although scientific research into this therapy is still thin on the ground, there are a few studies that suggest reflexology can help:

- alleviate stress and anxiety and improve feelings of well-being
- treat chronic headaches and migraines
- reduce the amount of pain relief needed after knee and hip surgery.

But none of these studies has been conducted as a properly controlled clinical trial, so the therapeutic effect claimed has not yet been proved.

A more rigorous study of the use of reflexology to treat pre-menstrual syndrome has found that those women who received reflexology experienced a much greater improvement in their symptoms than those women who did not.

What can reflexology do for you?

Reflexology is basically a good all-round therapy which aims to improve our general health and sense of well-being. However, reflexologists suggest that it can also help with various specific conditions such as:

- allergic problems, including hay fever and asthma
- aches and pains
- chronic conditions affecting children (e.g. colic and glue ear) and older people (e.g. confusion and dementia)
- detoxification
- digestive problems such as heartburn, constipation and diarrhoea
- headaches and migraines
- infertility, including low sperm counts in men and low ovulation in women
- the symptoms of jetlag
- menstrual problems, especially pre-menstrual syndrome
- pregnancy, labour and postnatal problems
- progressive disorders such as multiple sclerosis
- sinusitis
- skin problems like acne, eczema and psoriasis
- a weak immune system
- stress and anxiety
- tiredness and fatigue
- wound healing.

Reflexology in health care

Reflexology has become a very popular therapy within the health service, particularly among nurses – because it is relatively easy to learn, is pretty safe to use and requires no expensive or specialized equipment. It also seems to be effective. Areas in which reflexology has been used successfully include:

- in cancer care as a complement to conventional treatments
- on postnatal wards to help mothers and their babies recover after the birth
- on long-stay elderly care wards and in nursing homes to help with arthritis, stiffness, insomnia, agitation, skin conditions such as leg ulcers, and to help relief of mild depression
- in GPs' surgeries for the treatment of stress and stress-related problems.

Cautionary guidelines

Reflexology really is very safe to use, but reflexologists suggest that there are certain circumstances when it may not be appropriate. Here is a summary of the potential risks associated with reflexology.

Using reflexology safely

No adverse effects from reflexology have been recorded, but it still makes sense to follow these guidelines.

Safety tips for you

- Only practise reflexology when you are feeling well.
- Always wash your hands before and after a treatment.
- Make sure your nails are short and remove any rings, watches or bracelets that could get in the way.
- Make sure you are comfortable and avoid positions that could give you back or arm strain.

Safety tips for the person receiving reflexology (the receiver)

- Suggest a trip to the toilet before the treatment.
- Make sure the receiver is warm and comfortable.
- Clean and dry both feet thoroughly at the outset.
- Check for corns, calluses, swelling, deformities, in-growing toenails, and anything else that may be painful. Painful areas should be avoided. If severe problems exist, suggest a visit to a podiatrist.
- Check for cuts, bruises and foot injuries. Do not work on damaged areas.
- Check for health problems that might not be suitable for reflexology (see pages 12–13).
- Do not use creams, lotions or oils as they make it difficult to hold the foot properly, causing loss of leverage. If the receiver has perspiring feet, use a mild talcum powder.
- Explain to the receiver that, after the treatment, they may experience a 'healing crisis' (see page 12), but this a temporary reaction. If a problem continues, it may not be a healing crisis and medical advice should be sought.

The receiver may find it more comfortable to lie down while receiving treatment.

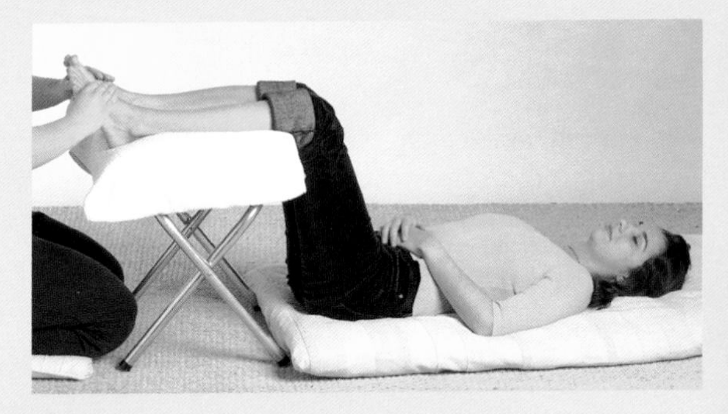

Safety in the treatment area

- Ensure the space you use is warm and clean.
- Check that the receiver will be able to sit comfortably with his or her feet supported in a raised position.
- Select a chair that is comfortable for you to work from.

Healing crisis

After the treatment, the receiver may experience a 'healing crisis', but this is a temporary reaction and should not last. Examples of healing crisis symptoms include:

- flu-like symptoms
- feeling light-headed
- feeling very cold for one to two days after a treatment
- increase in excretory functions
- reduction in blood pressure
- lethargy
- enhanced or altered sleep pattern.

When and how not to use reflexology

One of the most important rules is that you cannot make a diagnosis with reflexology. This needs to be explained to the receiver. The idea behind reflexology is to use observation and treatment therapeutically, regardless of what you or the receiver might think the problem is. It is also important not to promise to treat a specific problem. What you are working towards with reflexology is helping the body to seek its own equilibrium and produce a heightened sense of well-being.

Eunice Ingham (see page 5), one of the people who helped to develop reflexology, suggested that the only condition for which reflexology should not be used is thrombosis (blood-clotting within the veins). However, opinions vary. In the absence of thorough research, it is probably best to err on the side of caution! Here is a summary of the potential risks involved:

- During pregnancy – most reflexologists argue that reflexology is completely safe during pregnancy, but others suggest it is not suitable in the first trimester. It is certainly sensible to seek permission from the woman's doctor or midwife before offering a treatment.

- When a person has a pacemaker – they should get permission from their doctor before trying reflexology, and the chest area on the left foot should be avoided as it has been known for the pacemaker to move after treatment.

- For diabetics – reflexology is a balancing therapy and may well be beneficial to people with diabetes. However, it is always best to seek permission from the person's medical consultant before beginning any reflexology treatment.

- For depressive and manic states – someone who is psychotic, or taking large doses of psycho-active drugs, would probably not benefit from reflexology. It should also be used cautiously with anyone suffering from clinical depression.

- If renal (kidney) calculi or gall-stones are suspected – the renal reflexes, the gall bladder and the liver reflexes should be avoided as reflexologists have found that stones can move as a result of a treatment.

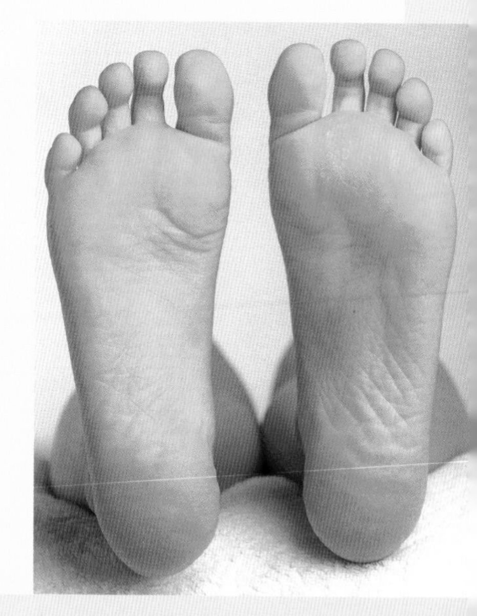

Theory *and* Practice

To use reflexology properly, you need to understand the principles that underpin it. This section offers a simple explanation of the theories involved. The techniques used in reflexology are easy to learn and the second half of this section includes simple, step-by-step instructions and practical tips.

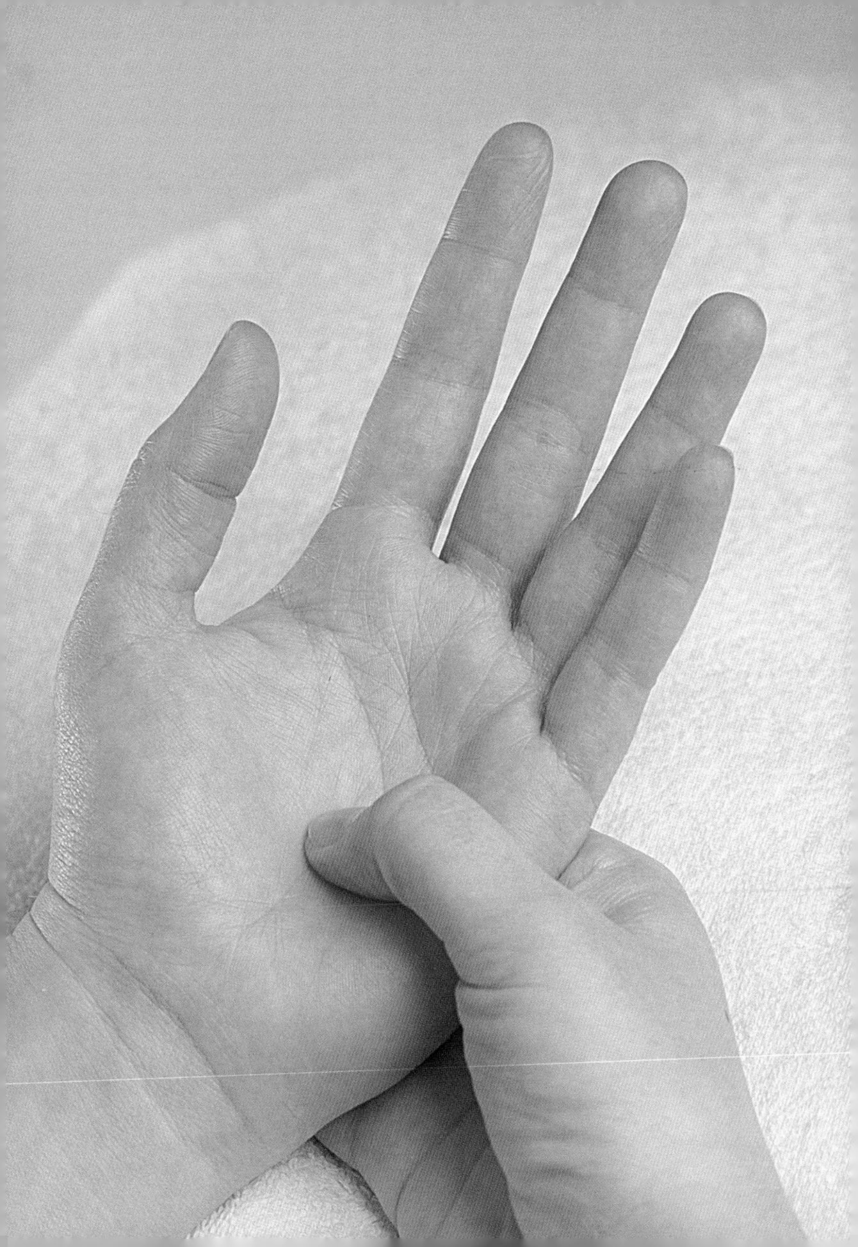

The principles of reflexology

Reflexology uses specific hand and finger techniques on reflex areas in the feet (and hands), which are said to correspond to particular organs and body parts. The theory is that these techniques cause a relaxation response in the part of the body represented by the reflex worked on. This in turn helps the body to return to a state of homeostasis (where all the body systems are maintained at equilibrium). Good health depends on the body's ability to return to homeostasis after an illness, a period of stress or an injury. So reflexology is seen as an aid to recovery and a way of maintaining good health.

Zone theory

The reflexes are said to be 'reflections' of the body parts and their location, and their relationships to one another are similar to those in the body. In fact, reflexology theory is based on the idea that the physical image of the body is projected on to the feet, and that this image is organized according to zone theory.

Zone theory is at the core of reflexology and is central to understanding it. The zones can be seen as markers which link one part of the body to another. There are 10 longitudinal zones, which run from the top of the head to the tips of the toes. Each finger and toe falls into one zone: the right thumb, for example, is in the same zone as the right big toe. The reflexes pass through the body within the same zones, so that the same point can be found on the front as well as on the back of the body, and on the bottom and top of the feet.

In reflexology, 'congestion' or tension in any part of a zone will affect the whole zone. If nothing is done, the congestion can spread to the areas on either side. Sensitivity in a particular part of the foot will tell a reflexologist where there is congestion in the body. The basis of zone theory is that direct pressure applied to any part of a zone will affect the entire zone. The reason the foot is mosty used in reflexology is because it is thought to mirror the body and to act as a terminus (end point) to the zones. Feet are also very sensitive to the touch.

There are also lateral or transverse zones on the body (see illustrations and table on pages 18–19). These are easily located and correspond to natural anatomical divisions. They help reflexologists to draw up a kind of grid system for the identification of reflex points.

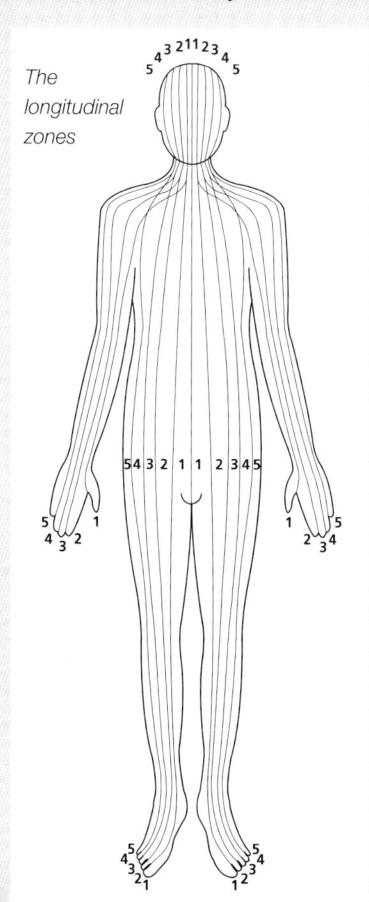

The longitudinal zones

The feet (and hands) should be seen as a pair and reflexologists look for the body's map in both feet at the same time. When studying the feet, certain points should be borne in mind:

- Each organ and body part can be found on the foot in the corresponding zone. The size of the reflex area within the zone often depends on the size of the corresponding organ.

- The reflex areas on the feet are sited according to the body's anatomy. For example, the heart is behind the lobe of the lungs.

- The right half of the body is reflected in the right foot, and the left half in the left foot. The only exception to this is the central nervous system, where the right half of the brain controls the left side of the body and vice versa. So, when the central nervous system has been affected, as in the case of a stroke, the reflexologist will work on the appropriate area of the foot on the opposite side from the trauma or injury.

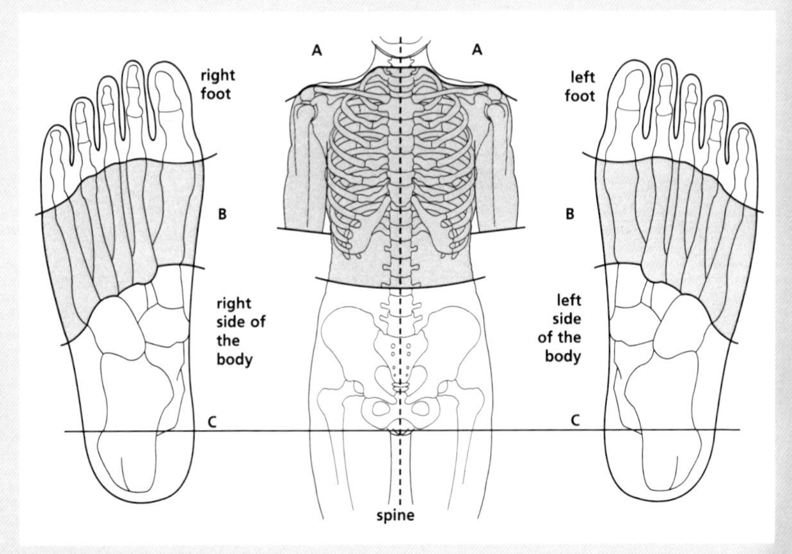

The transverse zones

Lateral zone	Location	Organ	Referral area on the foot
A	shoulder girdle	organs of the head and neck	toes
B	diaphragm	organs of the chest and upper abdomen	metatarsals Lisfranc's joint line
C	pelvic floor	organs of the abdomen and pelvis	tarsus, ankle joint

- Paired organs, like the lungs or kidneys, are to be found one in each foot. Single organs are to be found in either the left or the right foot, according to their anatomical position.

- The position of organs and body parts is also reflected in the zones of the feet, so that central organs such as the oesophagus are found on the inside of the feet and outer parts like the shoulder joint are found on the outside.

- The reflex areas of the organs are more easily accessible from the soles of the feet, whereas the nerves, muscles and bones are more easily treated from the top or back (dorsal side) of the feet.

An injured or painful area should never be worked on directly, but reflexology theory allows for this through what are called referral areas. These are different parts of the body that relate to each other through the zones (see box left) and are linked by body relation guidelines.

While reflexologists claim to have had excellent results from treating their clients according to zone theory, the mechanisms involved remain elusive. In the absence of any research into how reflexology works, people have variously suggested that the underlying mechanisms might be neurological, circulatory or perhaps involving the same sort of energy pathways that have been described in acupuncture and Chinese medicine.

Body area on foot	***Referral area on foot***
arm	leg
hand	foot
wrist	ankle
fingers	toes
shoulder	hip
upper arm	thigh
elbow	knee
forearm	calf

N.B. These relationships work in both directions. For example, if the thigh is injured, the referral area is the upper arm.

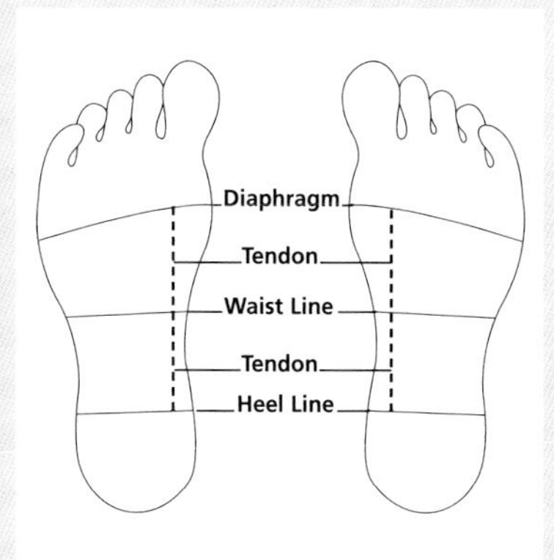

The four major body relation guidelines.

The feet – plantar view

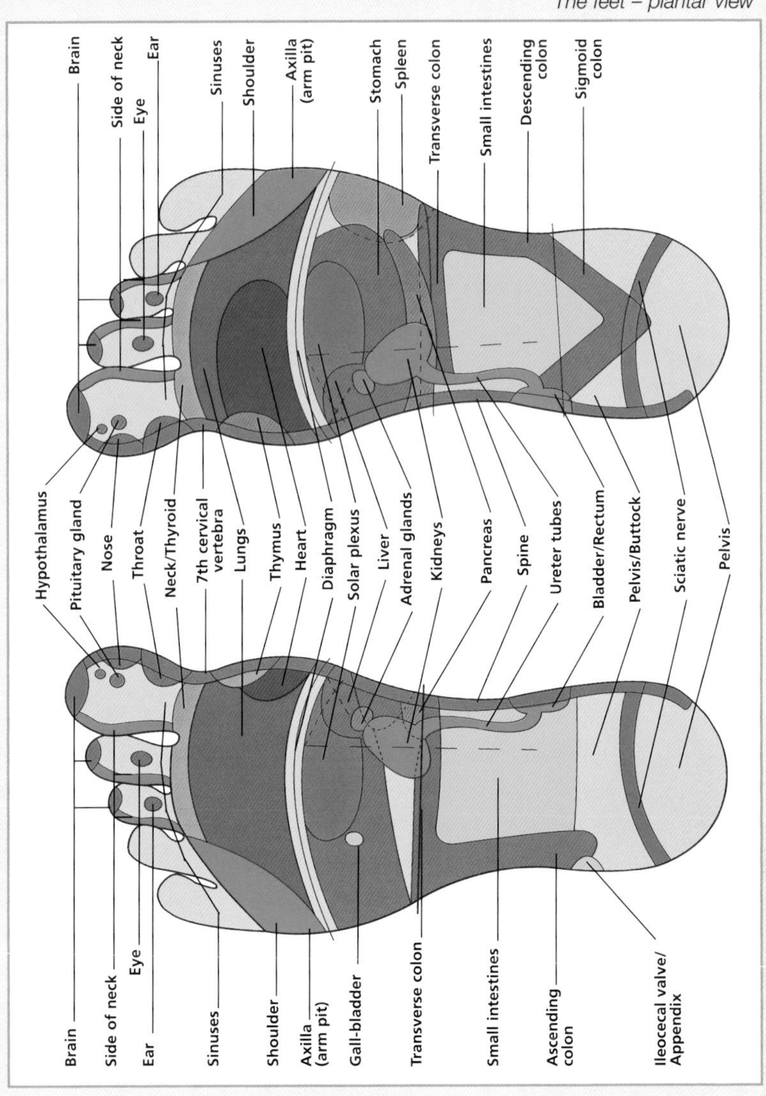

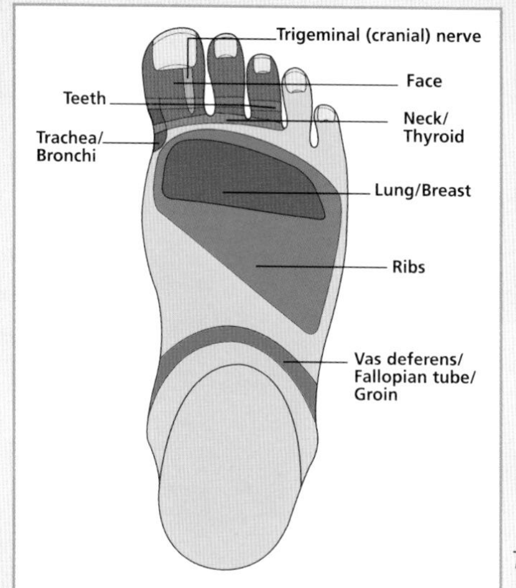

The feet – dorsal view

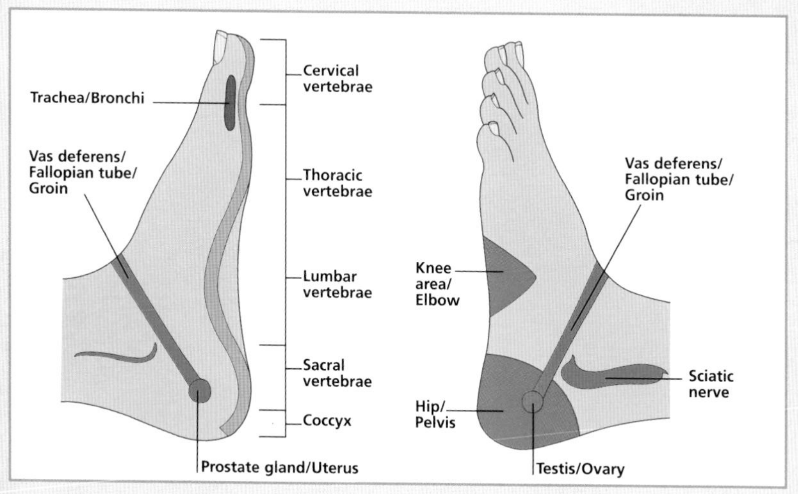

The feet – medial view

The feet – lateral view

The hands – Plantar View

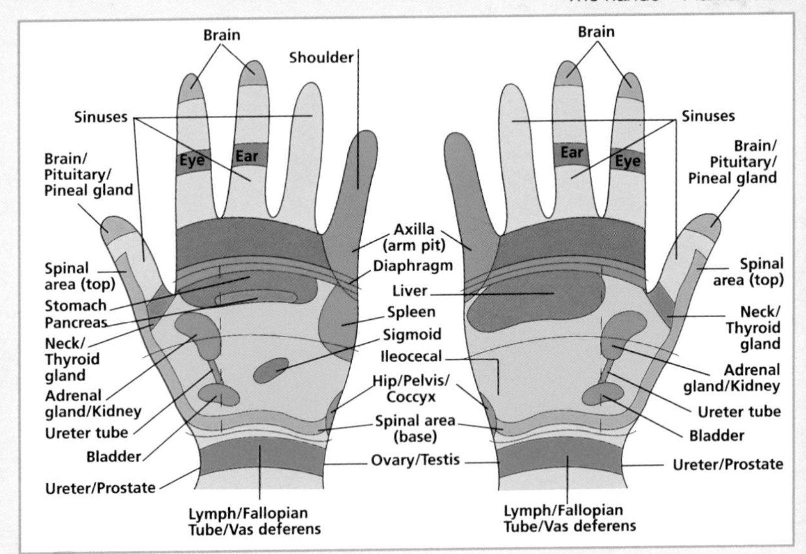

The hands – Dorsal View

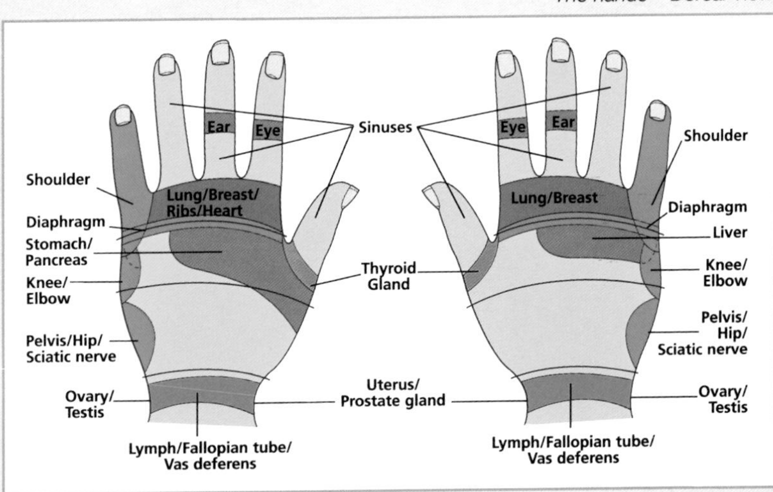

Learning reflexology techniques

The basis of reflexology technique is to work efficiently (i.e. with the least amount of effort to achieve the gain necessary) and to be effective (i.e. to find the right area to work on).

Good reflexology technique boils down to the correct use of the thumb and fingers. Key points to remember when practising reflexology include:

- The reflex points are tiny, so your thumb and finger movements need to be small and disciplined to achieve thorough coverage.

- The thumb and fingers should always move forwards, never backwards.

- Avoid circular movements or sliding.

- Never use the tip of your thumb or finger; always use the flat, pad part. To do this, your thumb or finger should not be too arched. This will ensure that your nails do not dig into the receiver's foot.

- When judging how much pressure to use, be guided by your intuition and the receiver's reaction – if he or she flinches, you are using too much pressure.

- The pressure applied should be smooth and consistent.

- A reflexology treatment should be an enjoyable experience for the receiver.

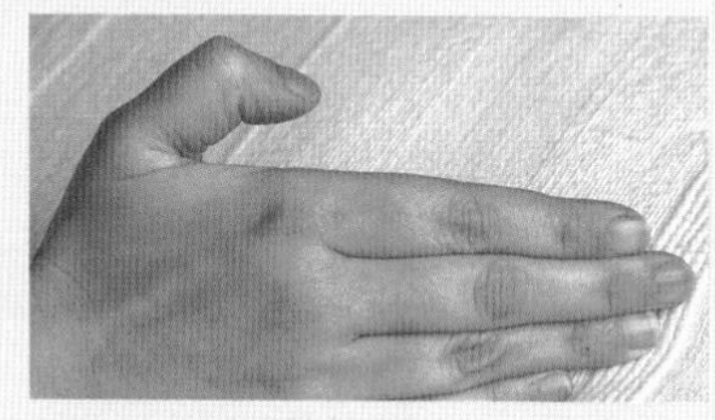

The thumb is too arched.

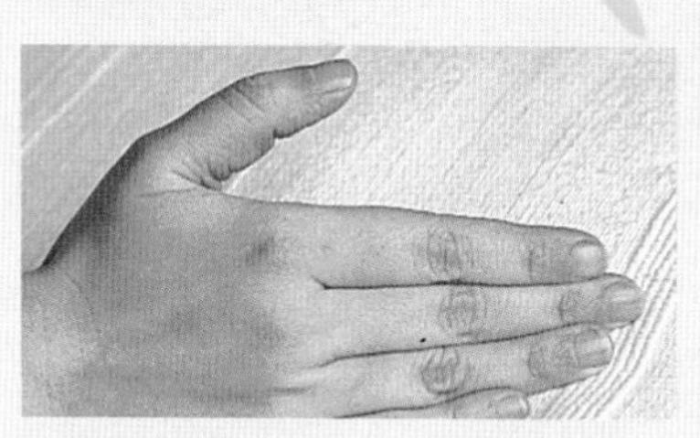

The thumb is too flat.

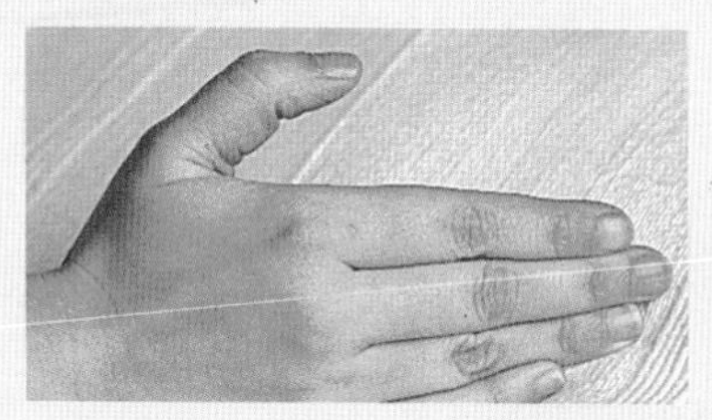

The thumb is at the correct angle.

The basic techniques

The techniques that follow are demonstrated on the foot, as this is the part of the body most commonly used in reflexology. Holding the foot correctly is essential to good reflexology technique. The hand that holds the foot is the 'holding hand', while the other is the 'working hand'.

There are three basic reflexology techniques:

- thumb walking – used to cover large areas
- finger walking – used for the tops and sides of the feet
- thumb hook and back-up – used to pinpoint specific points

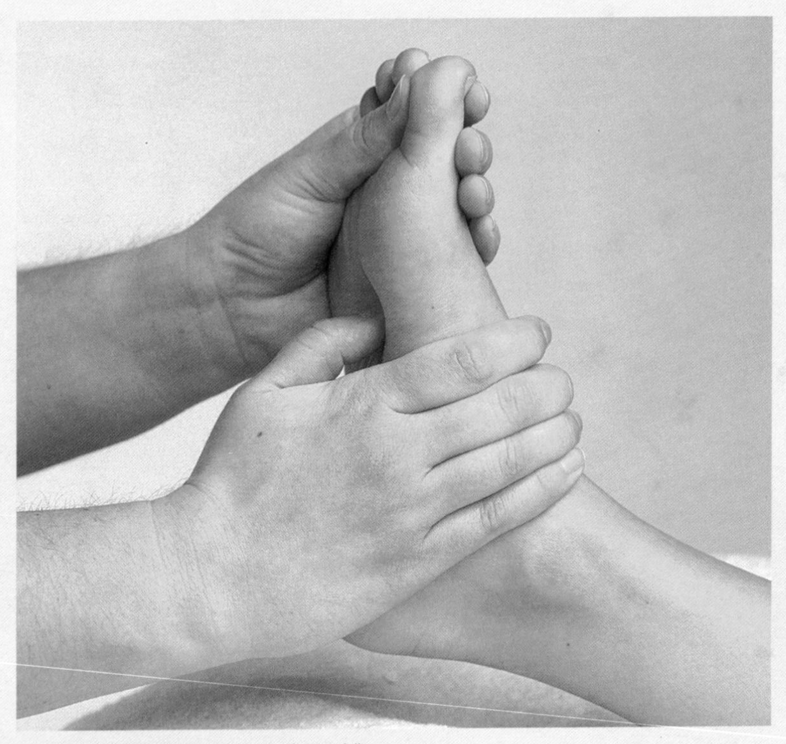

The holding hand supports the foot while the working hand gives the treatment.

Thumb walking

Sit comfortably and hold one of your thumbs below the first joint. Bend the first joint. Then try this exercise with your other thumb.

While still holding this thumb, place the outside corner of the thumb on your leg and bend the thumb at the first joint again (don't worry at this stage about how much pressure you are exerting, or what your other fingers are doing). To walk your thumb forward, allow it to rock forward on your leg from the thumb tip to the lower edge of the thumb nail. Remove your holding hand and unbend your working thumb, then bend and rock again. Do not push your thumb forward; it will move forward simply through the action of bending and unbending. Practise taking smaller 'steps'.

To make sure you have your thumb at the correct angle, lay your hands down on a flat surface. Feel where the thumbs rests on that surface, and walk them along the surface. It is this outside edge of your thumb that should make contact with the foot.

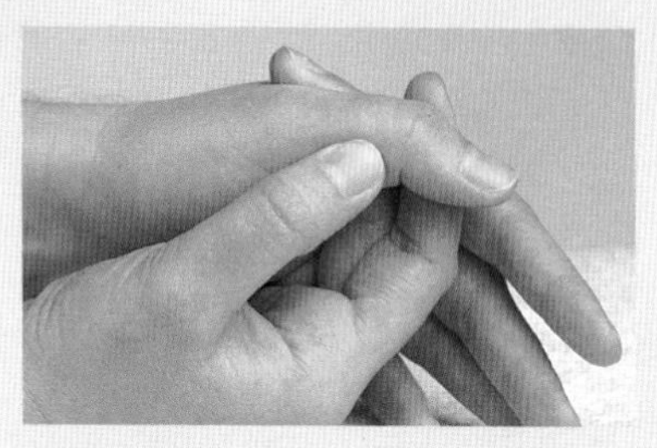

Hold one of your thumbs below the first joint and bend it.

Pressure in reflexology comes from the use of leverage, and in this technique leverage is attained by the use of the four fingers in opposition to the thumb. To get an idea of how this works, place the four fingers of your working hand on your opposite forearm. Press your thumb into the forearm. Now lower the wrist of your working hand, while keeping your fingers and thumb in position, and walk your thumb. With the wrist lowered, the pressure exerted by the thumb should have increased.

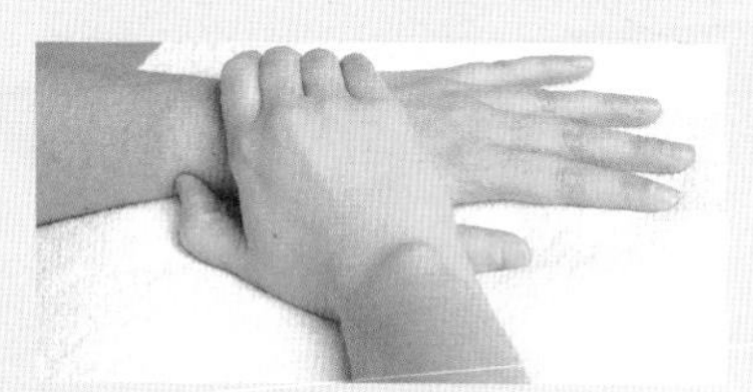

Lower your wrist to increase the pressure exerted by your thumb.

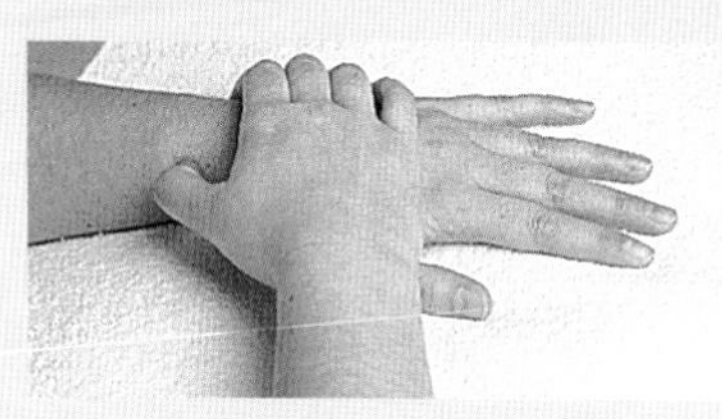

Raise your wrist to lower the pressure exerted by your thumb.

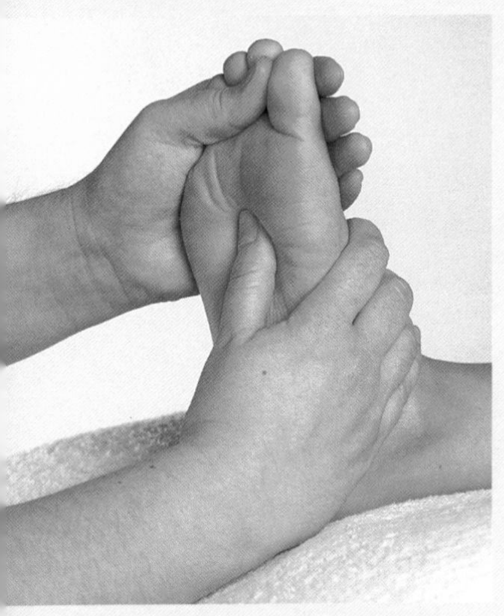

Your leverage fingers (of your working hand) should be contoured to the shape of the foot.

Constant pressure is essential when thumb walking and you will need to practise this technique regularly until you do not feel any on-off-on-off pressure at each bend of the thumb.

The next step is to try thumb walking on the feet, so you will need a willing volunteer to practise on!

Thumb walking is used to cover the large areas on the bottom of the foot. With your holding hand, grasp the toes, supporting them with your fingers, and gently hold them back to thin out the flesh and give the thumbs a chance to work on the reflex points. Practise walking the thumb of your working hand forward over the bottom of the foot. Ask your friend whether you are exerting a constant pressure. As you walk your thumb, check the position of your four 'leverage' fingers. Make sure they are together and in a natural hand position, contoured to the shape of the foot. As your thumb moves away from this natural hand position, you will need to reposition your leverage fingers accordingly.

Finger walking

This technique is very similar to thumb walking. This time, instead of using the thumb, you walk with the index finger of your working hand. Practise bending the first joint of your index finger in the same way as you did your thumb, then repeat with the tip of the finger resting on top of your holding hand.

'Walking' involves a slight rocking motion from the fingertip to the lower edge of the finger nail. As before, leverage is achieved by using your thumb in opposition to the fingers. To practise leverage, put the four fingers of your working hand on top of the opposite forearm. Press your fingers into your forearm and hold on with your thumb. Then raise the wrist of your

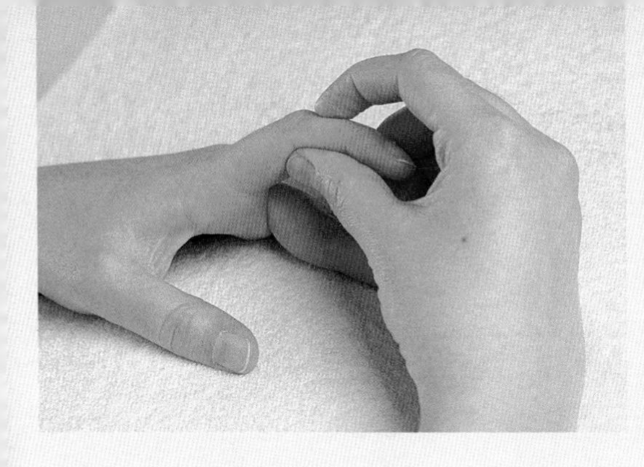

Practise the finger technique on your hands. As with thumb walking, the finger should always move in a forward direction, never backwards or sideways.

working hand and allow the index finger to walk. You can increase the pressure exerted by the index finger by raising the wrist and decrease it by lowering the wrist.

You should only walk one finger at a time, but it doesn't matter which finger you use – experiment and find out which one you feel most comfortable with. As your finger walks, allow the other fingers to move forward with it.

Thumb hook and back up

This technique is used to apply pressure to a particular point, rather than to cover large areas. This is called 'pinpointing'. Start by resting your thumb on the palm of your other hand. Bring your fingers up so that they touch the top of the hand and support it. Then bend the first joint of your thumb, exerting pressure in the same way as for thumb walking. Now pull the thumb back across the point. Leverage is attained in the same way as for thumb walking – lower the wrist to increase the thumb pressure.

Practise the technique for thumb hook and back up on the palm of your hand.

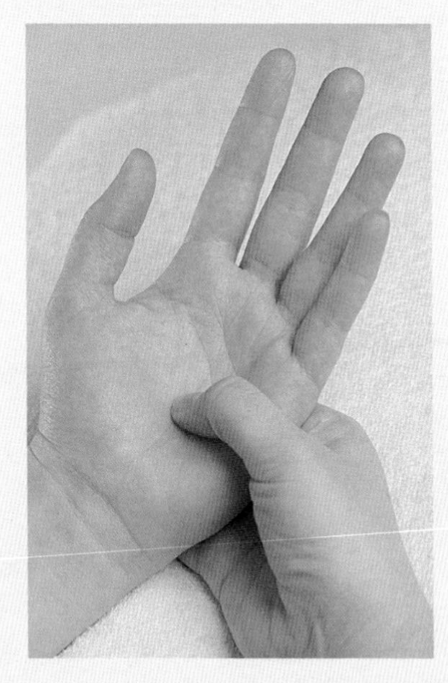

Giving a Treatment

Now you have learnt the basic techniques, you can put them together and create a relaxing reflexology treatment. This section offers advice on preparing your treatment area, making the receiver comfortable and preparing yourself to give a treatment. There are then some simple step-by-step guidelines for a foot treatment and suggestions for treating yourself with hand reflexology.

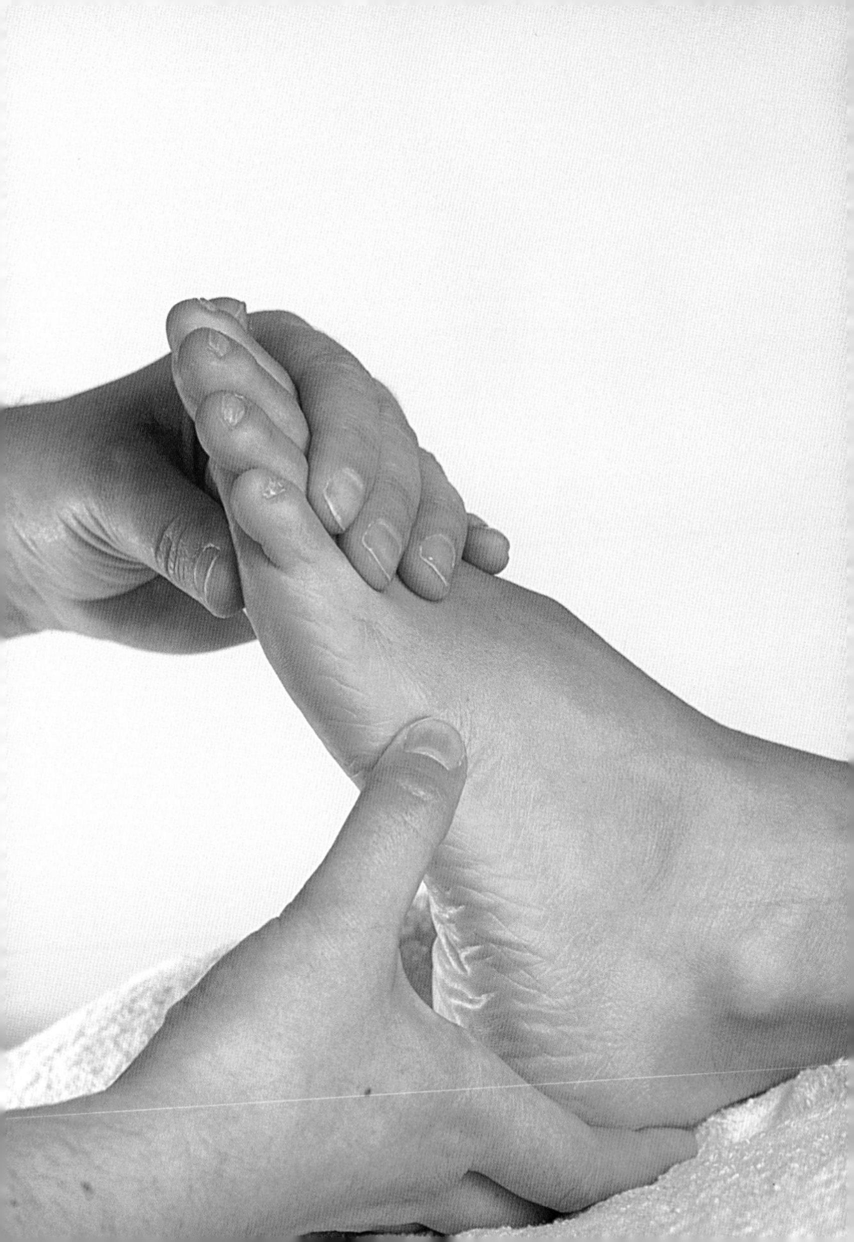

Preparation

To get the best out of a reflexology treatment it is important to be well prepared. This includes creating the right setting for the treatment as well as meeting the comfort needs of the person you are going to treat. You also need to prepare yourself so that you give the best treatment possible.

Preparing your treatment area

- Make sure the area is clean, tidy and draught-free, with room for you to work without feeling cramped. You will need a comfortable chair or sofa with a leg support that will allow the receiver's feet to be high enough for you to work without arm or back strain. A reclining chair or a garden lounger is ideal. Alternatively, you can perform the treatment on the floor, with the receiver's legs supported in a comfortable position. Keep a few cushions or towels to hand to make adjustments.
- Good lighting is necessary, but make sure it's not too harsh.
- Create a relaxing atmosphere with suitable music and a pleasant fragrance from fresh flowers, incense or perhaps a bowl of potpourri placed nearby.

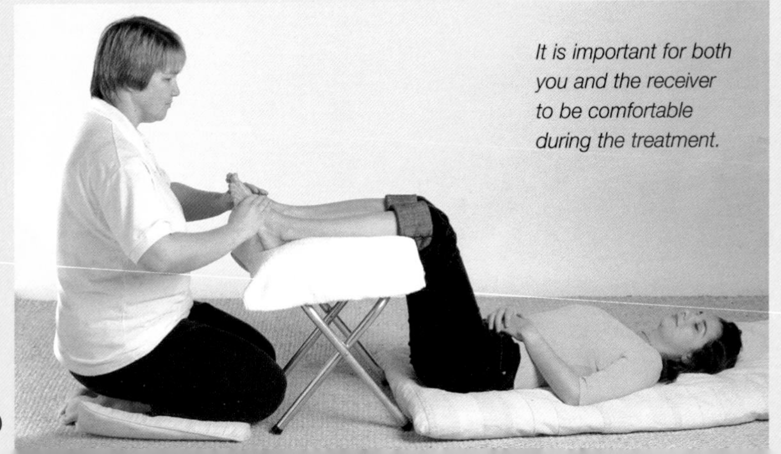

It is important for both you and the receiver to be comfortable during the treatment.

Preparing yourself

- Wear comfortable clothes with short sleeves or roll up long sleeves. Remove your watch and any rings or bracelets. Secure long hair away from your face. If the receiver is going to be seated, select a chair or stool for yourself that allows you to work without bending your back and to maintain eye contact with the receiver. Sit with both feet firmly on the ground. If the receiver is going to be on the floor, use a cushion to ensure that you are in the correct position.

- Ensure your hands are relaxed and supple. Holding a small rubber ball in one hand and alternately squeezing and relaxing your hand is one good exercise. Gently rotating and stretching each finger, as well as circling your wrists clockwise and anti-clockwise, is another.

- You should be relaxed and focused. Make sure you are breathing properly (breathe in slowly over a count of three or four, feeling your abdomen expand, then slowly breathe out), and take time to clear your mind. Sit quietly, breathe deeply and think about the receiver.

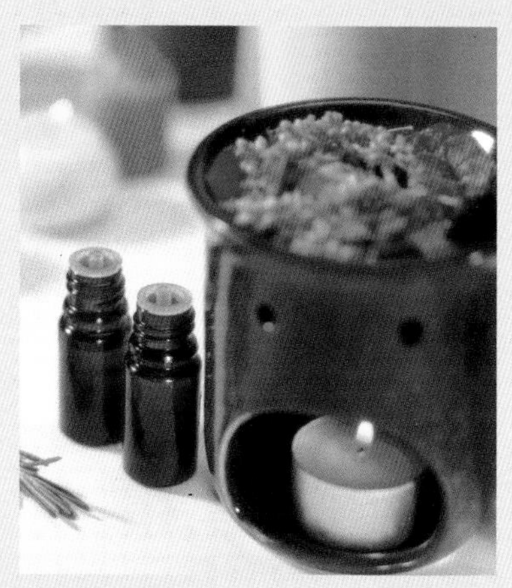

Choose a calming scent of potpourri or essential oil, such as lavender or jasmine.

- Wash your hands thoroughly before and after giving a treatment.

Making the receiver comfortable

- Ask the receiver to remove their shoes and socks or tights. Check that they are comfortable and use cushions to support them where necessary. If you are using a stool to support their legs, ensure it is cushioned and does not overly stretch the legs.

- Clean and dry the receiver's feet thoroughly before starting the session, and again afterwards.

Giving a foot reflexology treatment

A treatment session should take 40 to 50 minutes. If specific areas of the foot need more attention, the session can last up to an hour.

The following sequence is fairly standard, though each reflexologist has his or her own chosen routine and technique. Having said that, most reflexologists would consider this to be a thorough sequence.

Points to bear in mind include:

- work each foot twice
- keep at least one hand on the foot at all times
- always start a treatment with the same foot.

1 Before you start, check for anything that might be painful to the touch. Ask the receiver about any problems.

2 **Side to side (relaxation technique)**
Place your hands on either side of the foot and move it back and forth – when the right hand moves away from you, the left hand comes towards you, and vice versa. It is a rapid rocking motion, but try to keep your hands relaxed.

3 **Hook in the ankle (relaxation technique)**
Hook the base of both palms just above the back sides of the heel so that the palms lie next to or cover the ankle bones. As with Side to side, use an alternating motion with your right and left hands to work the foot from side to side. The foot should wiggle back and forth in an almost blurred motion. As before, try to keep your hands relaxed.

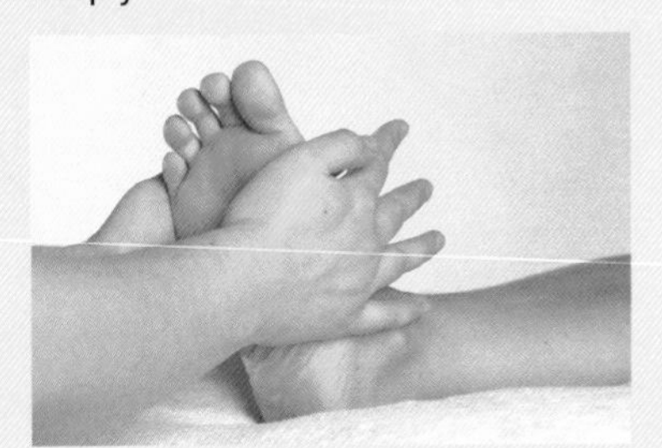

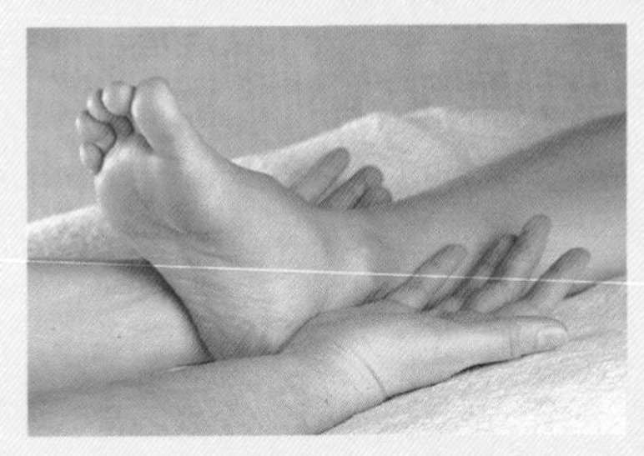

4 Rotating the ankle (relaxation technique)

Grasp the right foot around the ankle with your right hand (or the left foot with your left hand). Wrap your fingers round the heel so that the thumb rests in the lymphatic area. With your other hand, hold the inside of the foot below the base of the big toe. Use even pressure with both hands and rotate the foot smoothly in 360° circles in both directions.

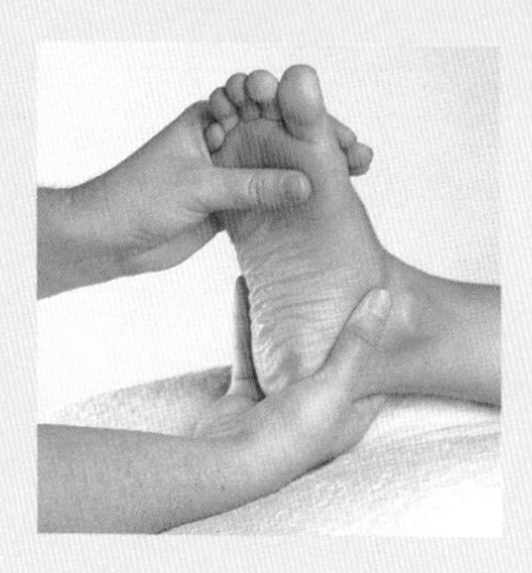

5 Spinal twist (relaxation technique)

Place your hands around the foot so that the index fingers are next to each other on top of the foot, while the thumbs are together on the bottom of the foot. Use a wringing motion with the hand nearest the toes, keeping the other hand still. Then re-position your hands so that they are both slightly closer to the toes and wring again. Repeat as often as you like. The idea is to twist the foot around the spinal area, not to twist the whole foot.

6 Lung pressure (relaxation technique)

Make a fist (with your right hand for the right foot, and left for the left foot), and place it on the bottom of the foot in the lung area. Curve your other hand around the top of the foot across the lung area. Press your fist against the foot, using the other hand as a backstop. As you reduce the pressure, squeeze with your other hand and push with it back towards the fist, which acts as the backstop. These two movements should be wave-like.

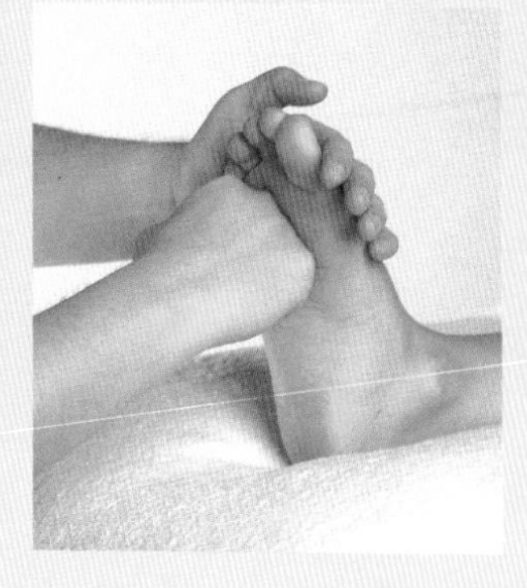

7 Solar plexus/diaphragm (relaxation technique)

Use thumb walking to work the area. Hold the toes back with your holding hand. Place the fingers of the working hand on the top of the foot for leverage.

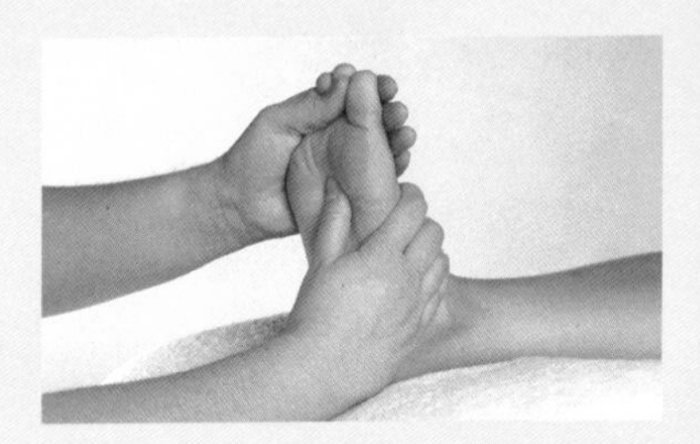

8 Seventh cervical

Anchor the big toe with the thumb and fingertips of your left hand. Place the other thumb on the bottom of the toe and walk your finger all around the base of the big toe.

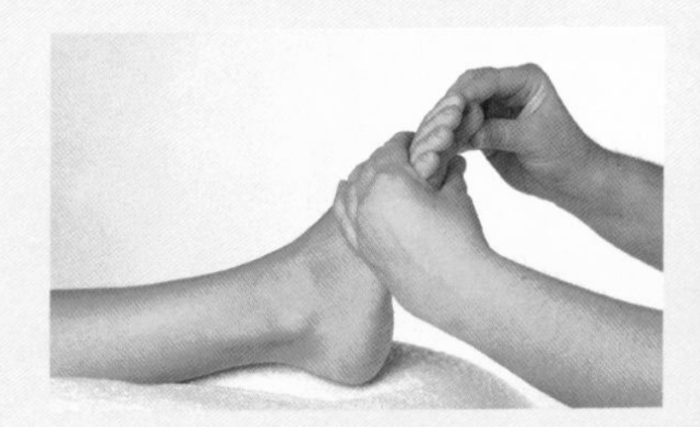

9 Thyroid/parathyroid

Use your holding hand to support and protect the big toe, and the thumb to hold it. Place the fingers of your working hand on those of the holding hand. Use thumb walking over the area. Change hands and walk from the other direction.

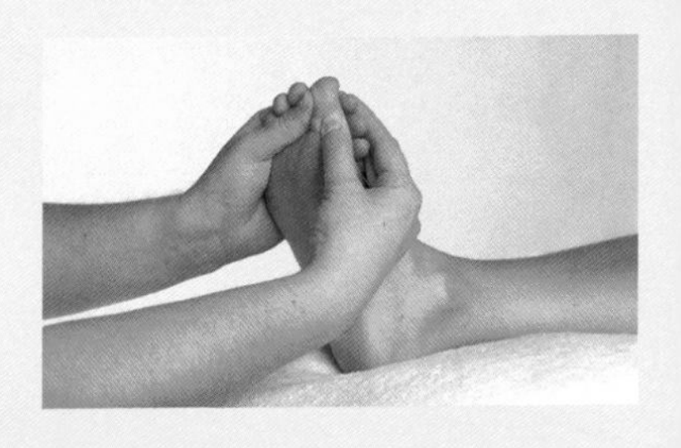

10 Pituitary

Look for the widest point on the big toe. Draw an imaginary line between these points – the pituitary lies on its midpoint. Support the big toe with your holding hand. Place the fingers of your working hand on top of the holding hand. Then place your thumb just beyond the pituitary point and use the hook and back-up technique.

11

Top of head

Anchor the big toe with the thumb and fingers of your holding hand. Join the thumb and index finger of the working hand and, using the thumb as support, roll the end of the index finger across the tip of the big toe, exerting a downward pressure. Then reposition your index finger and thumb and repeat until the whole of the tip of the toe has been covered. Repeat on the other toes.

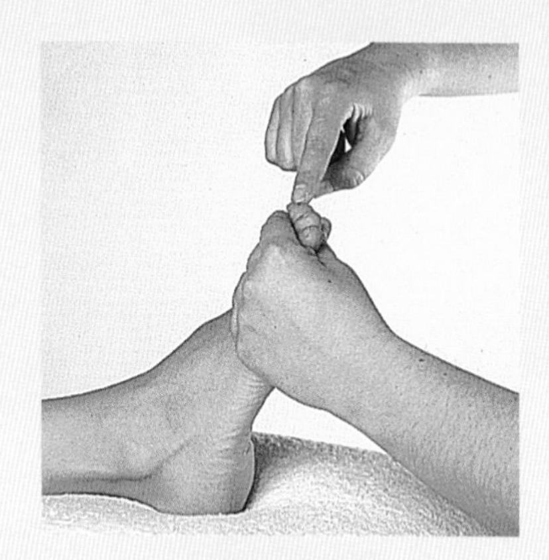

12

Toe rotation (relaxation technique)

Place the fingers of your working hand on the big toe as shown. The fingertips should extend almost to the base of the toe. Exert firm, even pressure with the grasping fingers, and pull upwards slightly. Rotate the toe slowly and evenly in both directions. Repeat with each toe.

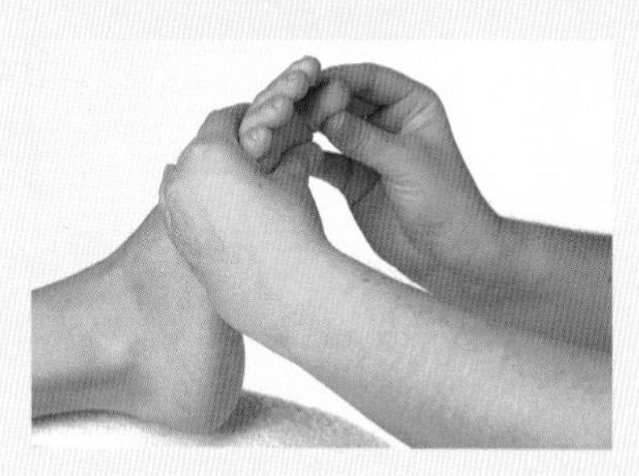

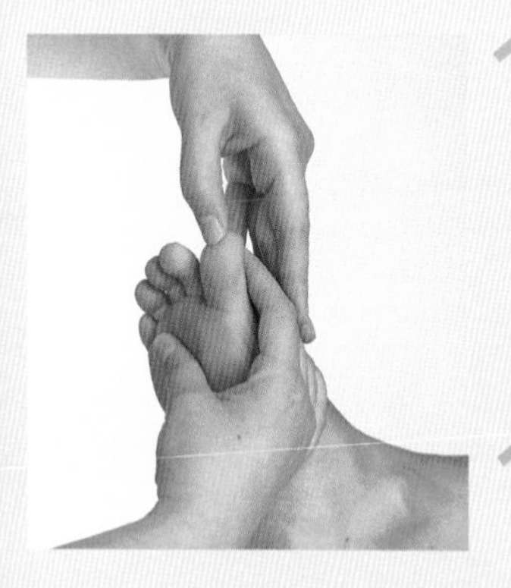

13

Head/neck/sinus (big toe)

Support and protect the big toe with your holding hand. Place the fingers of your working hand on the fingers of the holding hand. Use thumb walking to walk down the centre and along each side of the toe. The holding fingers act as a backstop throughout.

14

Head/neck/sinus (small toes)

Repeat 13 for each of the small toes.

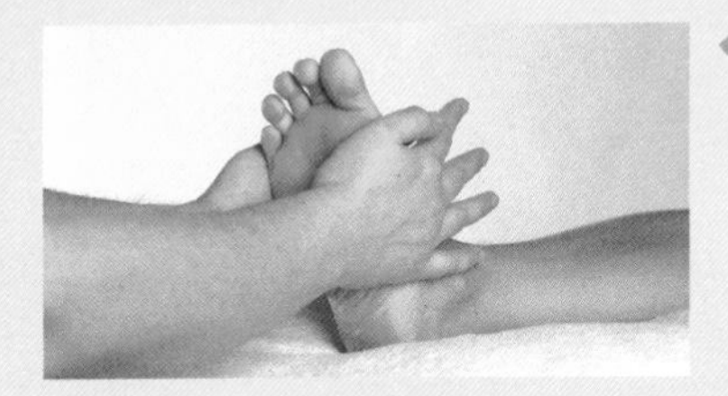

15 **Side to side**

Repeat 2.

16 **Ear/eye**

Use the holding hand to pull the pad of the foot down to open the area up. Using thumb walking along the top of the ridge, exert downward pressure towards the heel along the top of the ridge. Change hands and walk across the ridge from the opposite direction.

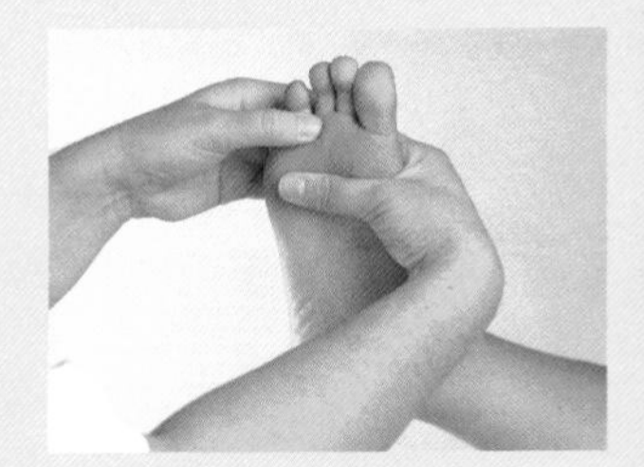

17 **Head/neck/sinus (top of toes)**

Use the thumb of your holding hand to support the toe you are working on. Start at the top of the toe and use finger walking down each side and along the centre of the top of each toe.

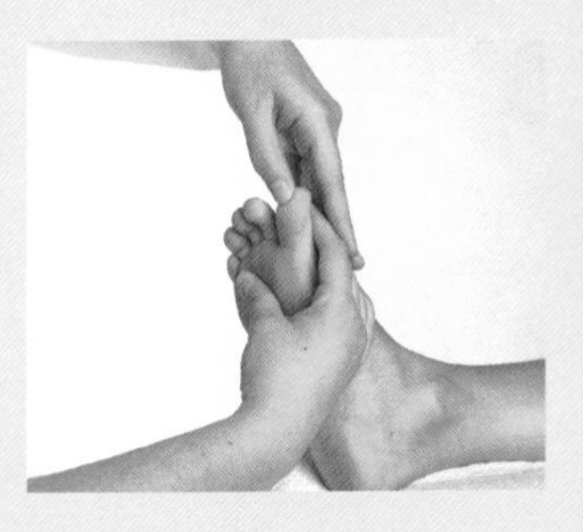

18 **Lung**

To widen the troughs running across the top of the foot, spread the toes apart using the fingers of your holding hand as a relaxed fist under the foot. Use the thumb of your working hand to push on the ball of the foot and use the index finger to walk down each trough. If needed, use the middle finger to support the index finger.

19 Lung

Hold the toes of the right foot back with the left hand (or left foot with the right hand) and walk the four troughs between the toes on the ball of the foot using your thumb. Change hands if you find you are stretching your thumb too much to reach the furthest troughs.

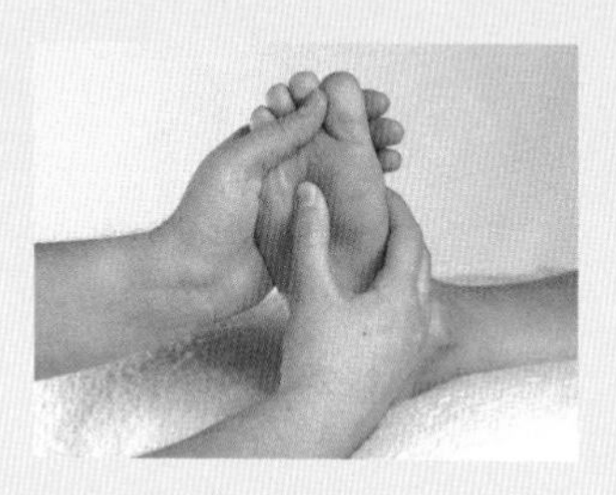

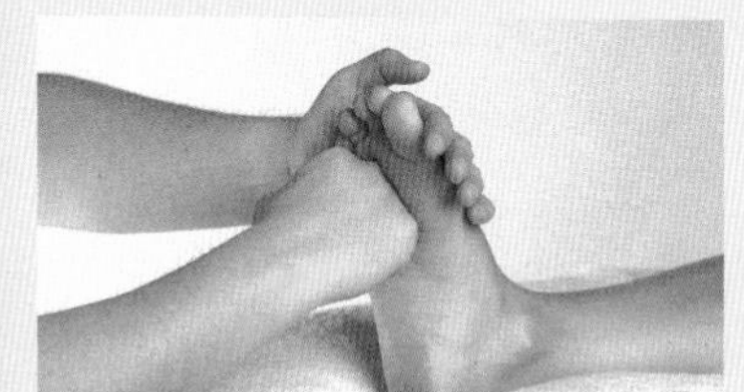

20 Lung pressure

Repeat 6.

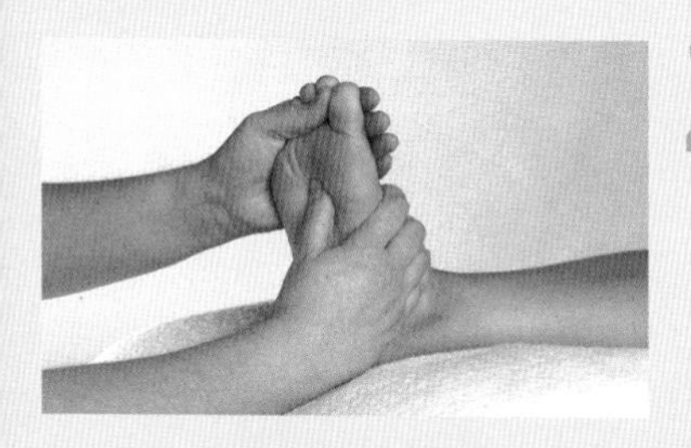

21 Solar plexus/diaphragm

Repeat 7.

22 Arm

Hold the right foot with the right hand (or the left with the left hand). Place the fingers of your left hand on the top of the foot and walk the thumb of your right hand around the outside of the foot several times. Change hands to walk the area from the other direction.

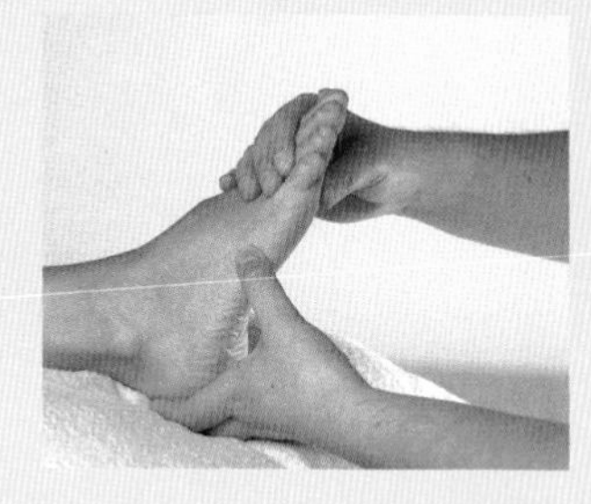

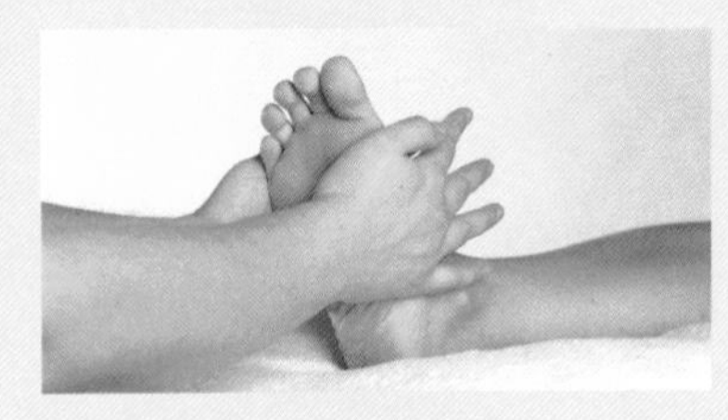

23 Side to side
Repeat 2.

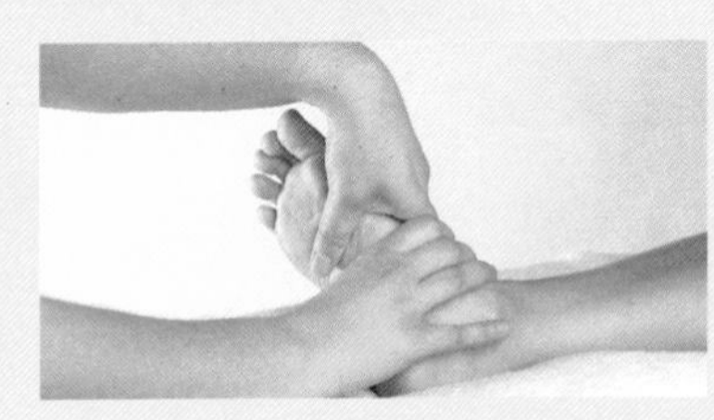

24 Spinal twist
Repeat 5.

25 Above the waistline
The waistline is an imaginary line across the foot from the fifth metatarsal, which is midway down the outside of the foot. Thumb walking is used to work all of the reflexes in this area. Use the left hand to hold the right foot (or the right hand to hold the left). Start from the waistline on the inside of the foot tendon and thumb walk along the tendon to the adrenal glands area. Then work diagonally across this area. Change hands. Walk the other thumb diagonally across the area. Repeat.

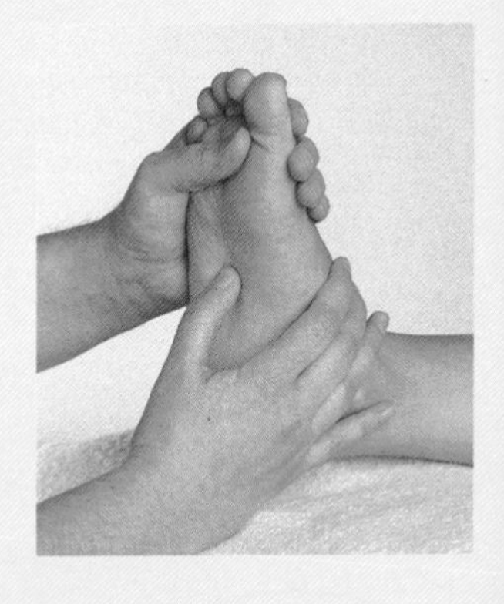

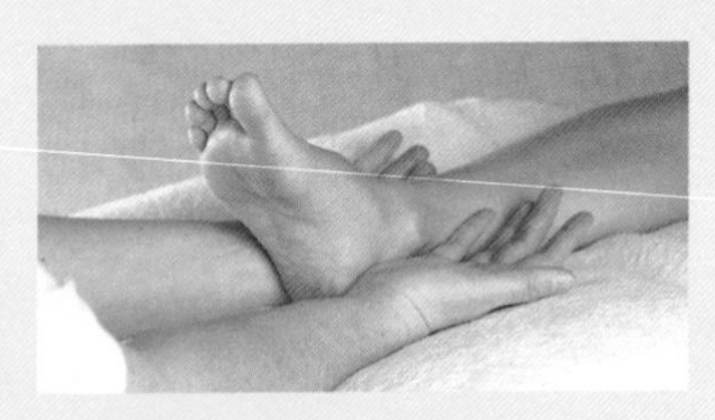

26 Hook in the ankle
Repeat 3.

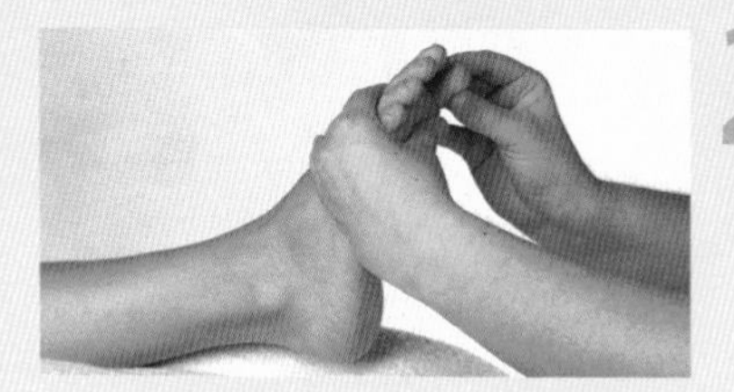

27 Toe rotation
Repeat 12.

28 Ileocecal valve (right foot)
The ileocecal valve lies between the small and large intestine areas. Run your hand down the outside of the foot from the fifth metatarsal bone to the heel. The valve is located in the deepest part of the hollow. Use the hook and back up technique.

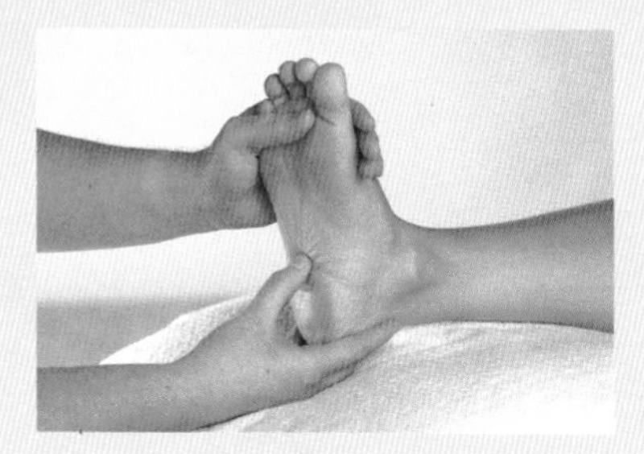

29 Below the waistline
Repeat 25, but cover the area below the waistline down to the beginning of the heel.

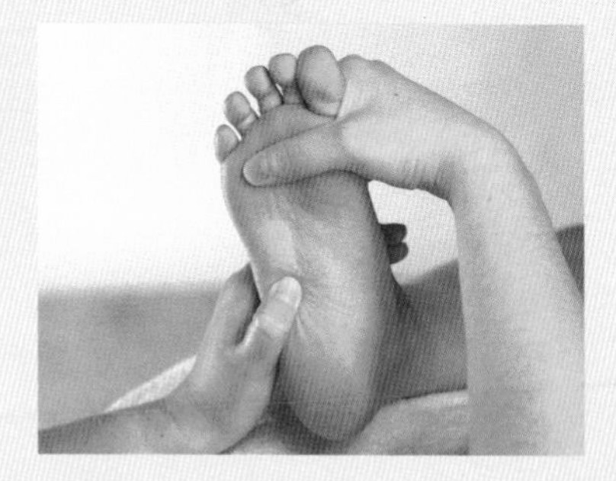

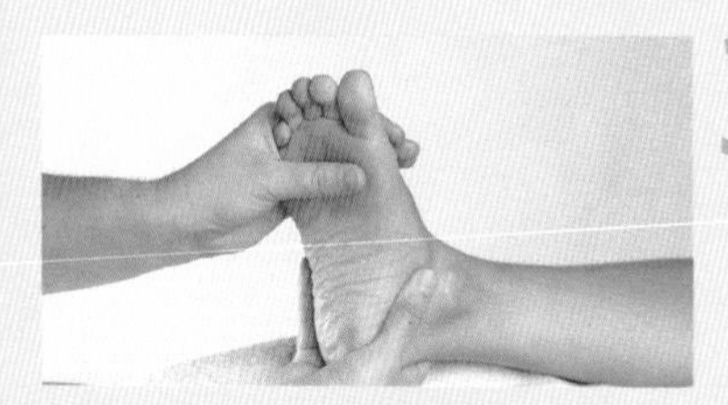

30 Rotating the ankle
Repeat 4.

31 Tailbone
Support the right foot in your left hand (or the left in your right hand). Thumb walk in a criss-cross pattern over the area from the bottom of the heel upwards.

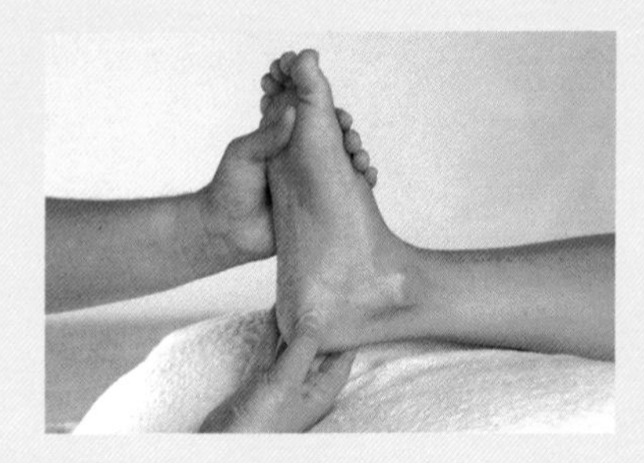

32 Back
To work the spine, thumb walk up along the spine area from the tailbone area. You can use the thumb walking technique from several directions, and finger walking as well.

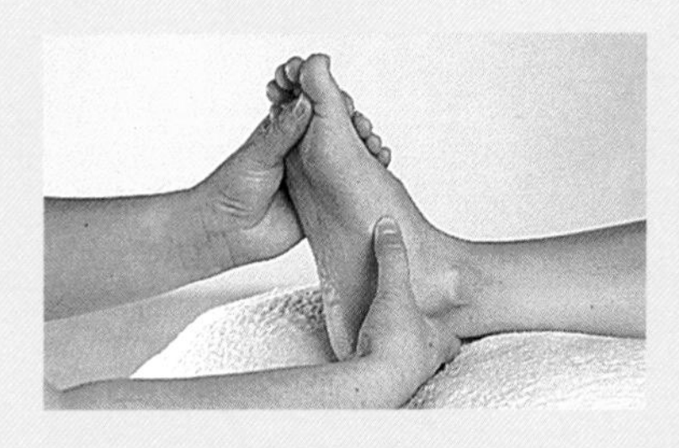

33 Spinal twist
Repeat 5.

34 Hip/back/sciatic nerve
Use finger walking around the outside ankle bone, while cupping the left foot with your right hand (or the right with your left hand). Then cup your right hand under the ankle and heel and finger walk from the top of the foot down to around the ankle bone.

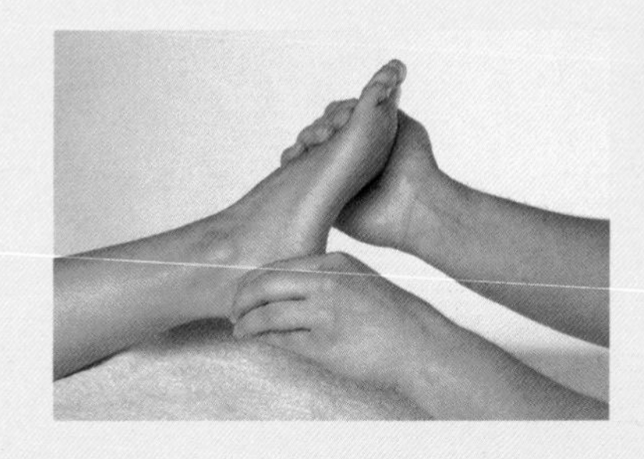

35

Hip region

The area involved is located on the inside and outside of the foot. Cup the working hand around the back of the ankle and finger walk down the area.

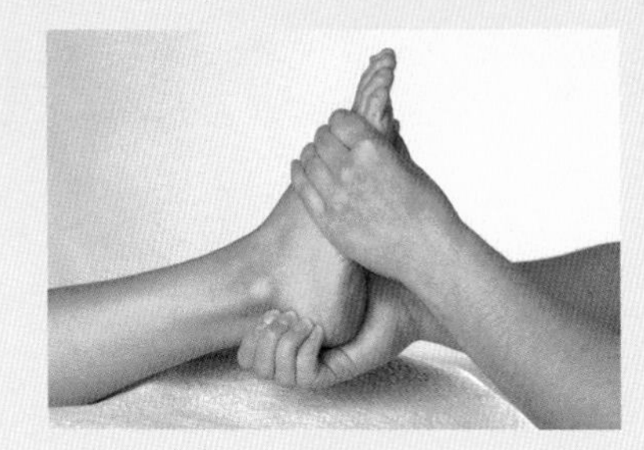

36

Knee/leg

The area on the foot for the knee and thigh is bordered by the fifth metatarsal, the front edge of the heel on the bottom, and the bony area on the side of the foot. Work this area several times either with thumb or finger walking.

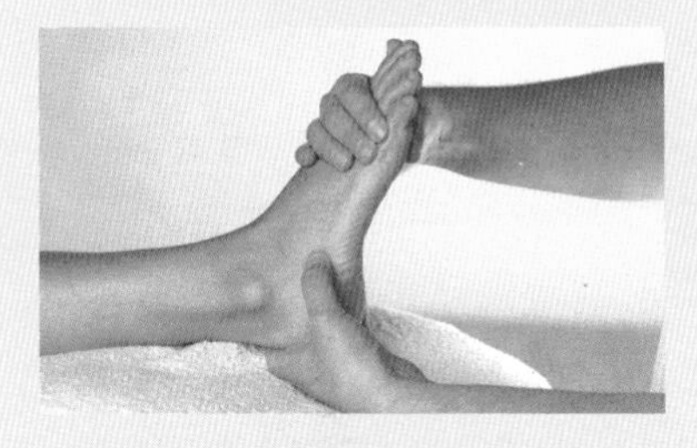

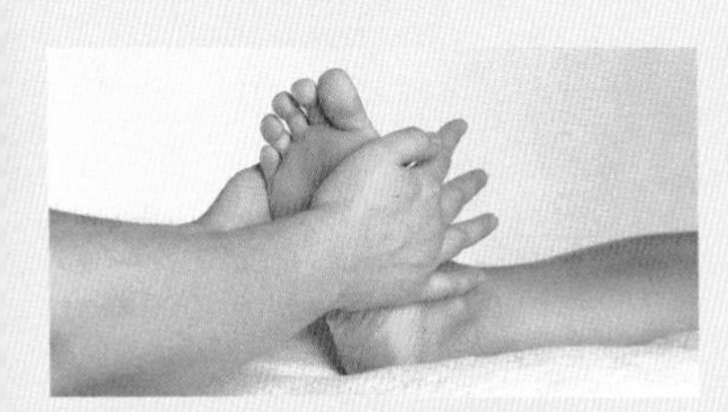

37

Side to side

Repeat 2.

38

Ovary/testicle

Walk the area located on the bony outside of the foot with the thumb of your left hand for the right foot (or of the right for the left foot).

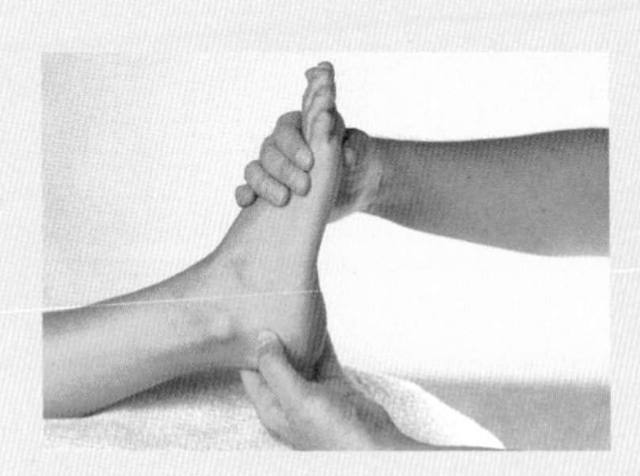

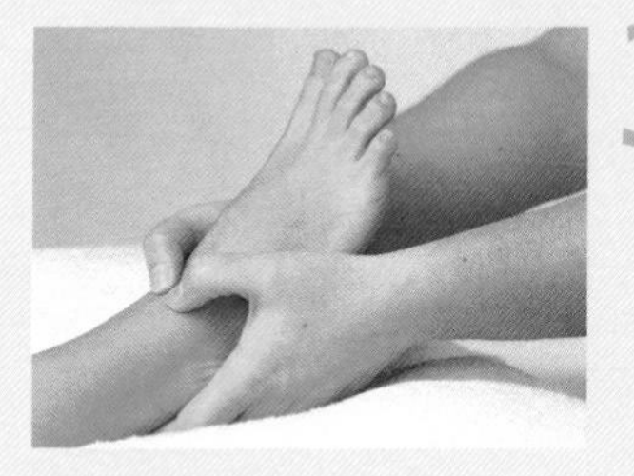

39 Lymphatic

This area stretches from the inside ankle bone around the top of the foot (crease) to the outside ankle bone. To work with the thumb, wrap the fingers of your working hand around the ankle and walk with the thumb along the crease. To work in the opposite direction, swap hands.

40 Uterus/prostate

This area is located on the inside of the foot below the ankle bone. To find it, place your index finger on the ankle bone and your fourth finger on the back of the heel. Place your third finger on the midway point – this is the reflex you need. Cup the right heel in your left hand (or vice versa), curling your third finger so its tip is on the reflex point. The thumb should be in the lymphatic area on the top of the foot. Rotate the foot several times with your other hand in both directions. Vary the pressure exerted by your finger, but be guided by the receiver's reaction. To link the prostate to the testis or uterus to the ovary, place the third finger of each hand on the reflex point on each side of the foot and rotate the finger gently – it will feel as if there is a rod through the foot.

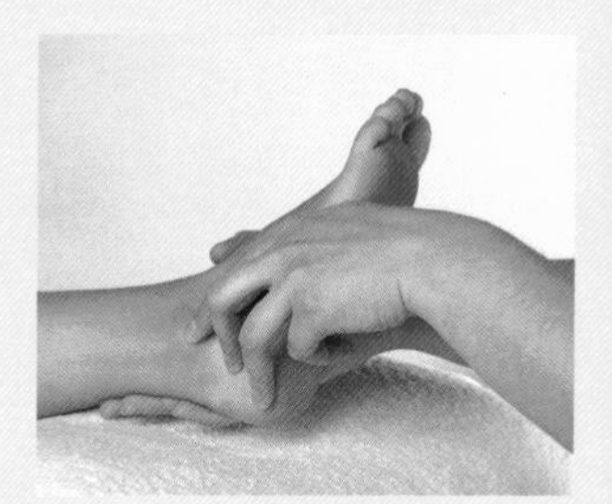

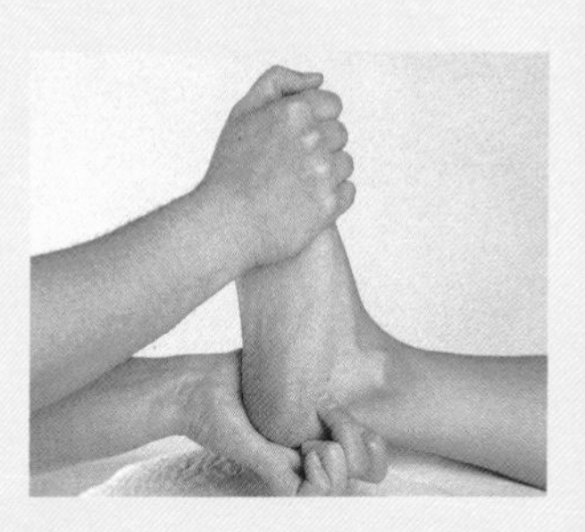

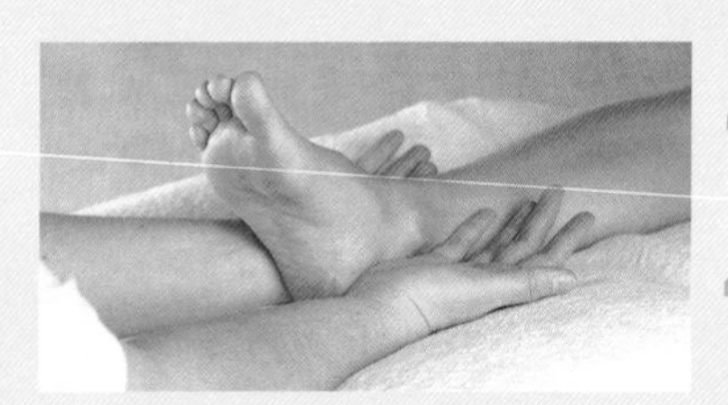

41 Hook the ankle

Repeat 3.

42 Repeat 2–41.

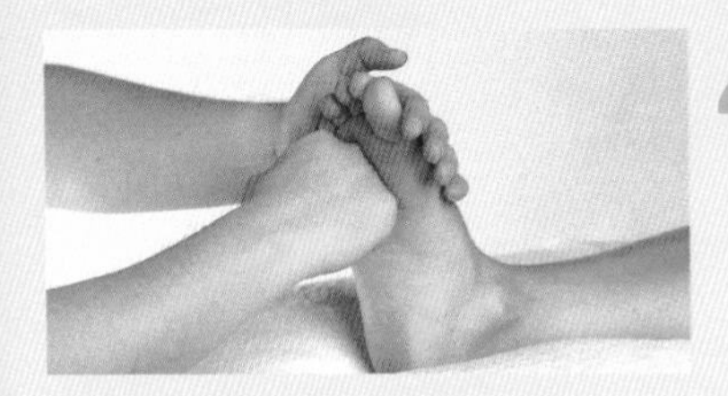

43

Lung pressure
Repeat 6.

44

Feathering (relaxation technique)
This is a light, rhythmic movement using the thumb walking technique over the solar plexus/diaphragm area. Feathering can be used on all parts of the foot as a relaxation technique during a treatment.

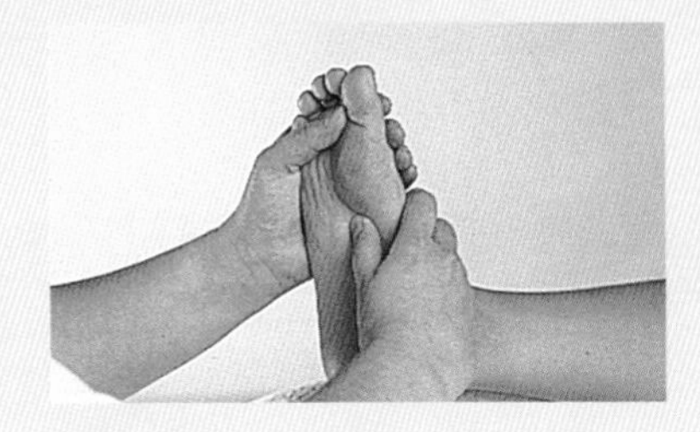

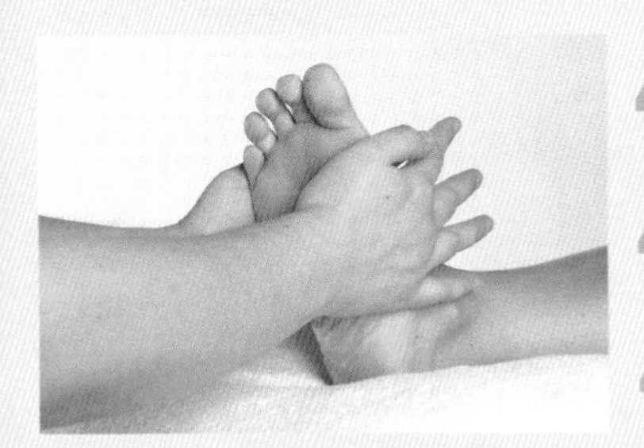

45

Side to side
Repeat 2.

46

Follow the sequence 2–42 for other foot.

47

Follow the sequence 43–45 for other foot.

48

Solar plexus exercise (relaxation exercise)
Take both feet and place the fingers of each hand on the tops of the feet. Position each thumb in the hollow between the big toe and the second toe, below the ball of the foot. Ask the receiver to take four deep breaths, while you exert a gentle, straight inward pressure with both thumbs. Gradually release the pressure on the last exhalation.

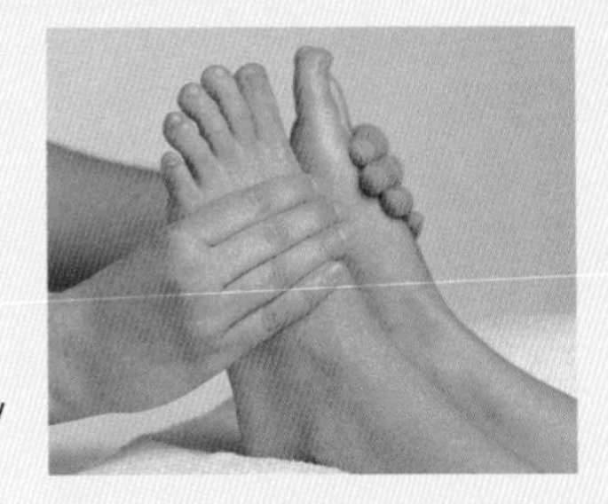

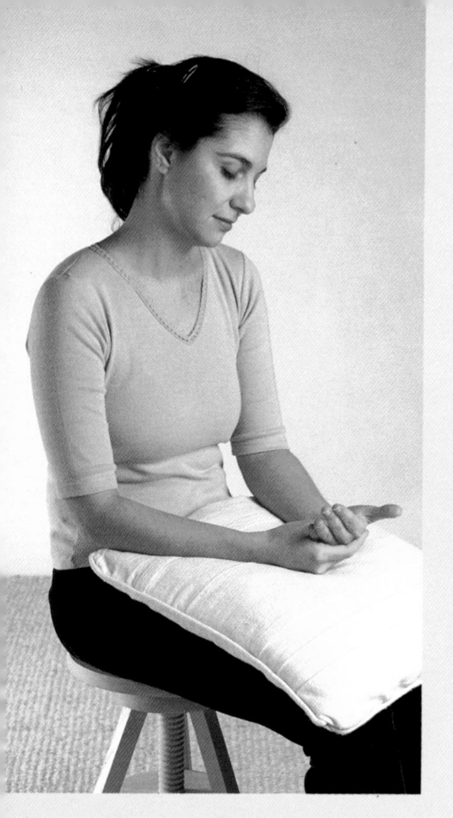

Treating yourself

It is extremely difficult to practise reflexology on your own feet. If you wish, you can, however, purchase various reflexology shoes, mats, rollers and brushes that are said to stimulate the reflexes and are designed for self-help purposes.

A limited form of hand reflexology on yourself is possible. You will need to sit comfortably with the hand to be treated, supported by the other hand, on a small cushion on your lap.

Spend about 10 minutes working on each hand using the sequence on the following pages. Start with the right hand, then work on the left. If you find a particularly sore area, it is worth working on that part of your hand again.

1 Lungs
Support your right hand with the fingers of your left hand. Walk your left thumb up from the diaphragm line of your right hand to where the fingers meet your palm. When you have finished walking your thumb, walk your left index finger down about 2cm (3/4 inch) from the point where the fingers join the hand.

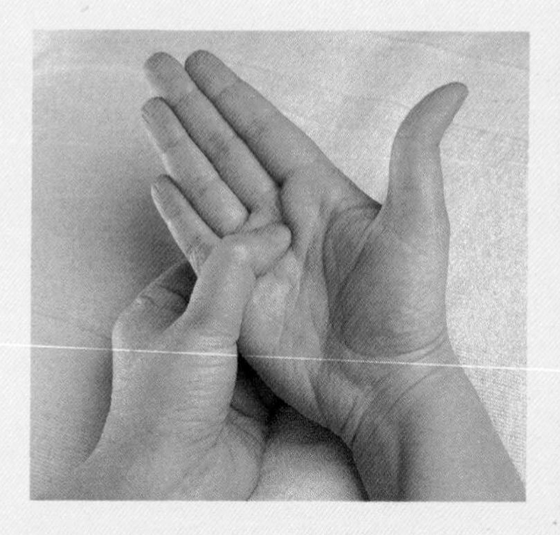

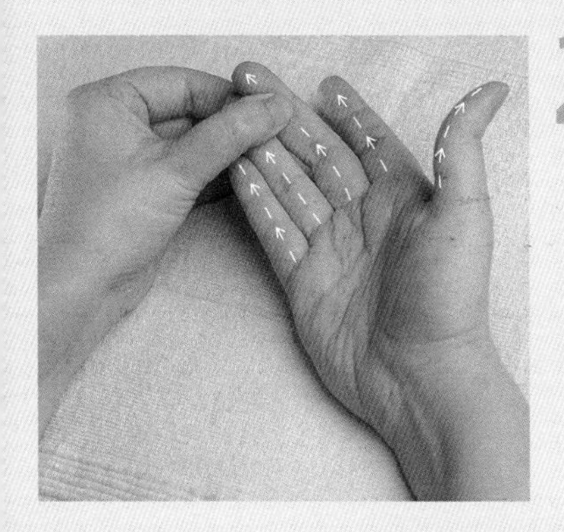

2 Sinuses

Walk the thumb of your left hand up the reflex points along the centre of each finger and thumb, starting at the palm and going up to the fingertip.

3 Eyes and ears

Exert pressure on the first joint of the index finger of your right hand, using your left thumb. Repeat for the first joint of your third finger.

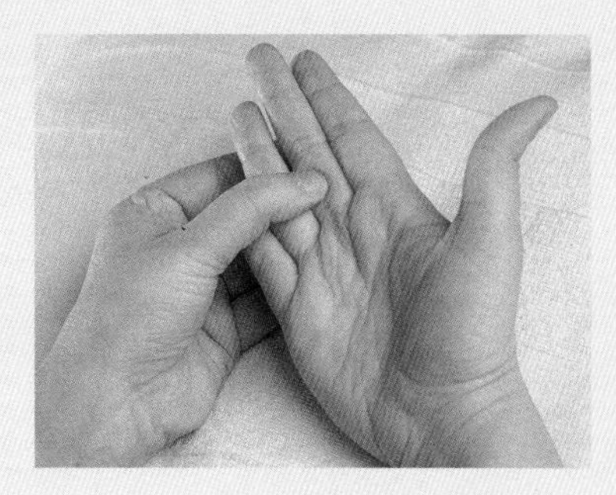

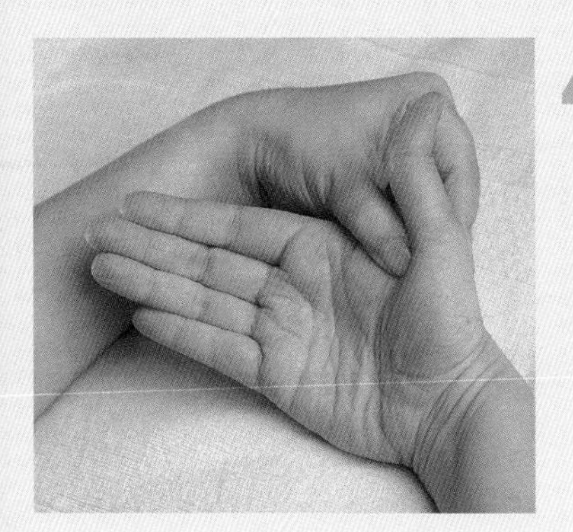

4 Neck and thyroid gland

Use the thumb hook and back up technique to pinpoint the reflex points at the base of your thumb and the first two fingers of your right hand.

5 Hip, knee and leg

Use the four fingers of your left hand to exert pressure around the lateral side of your right hand.

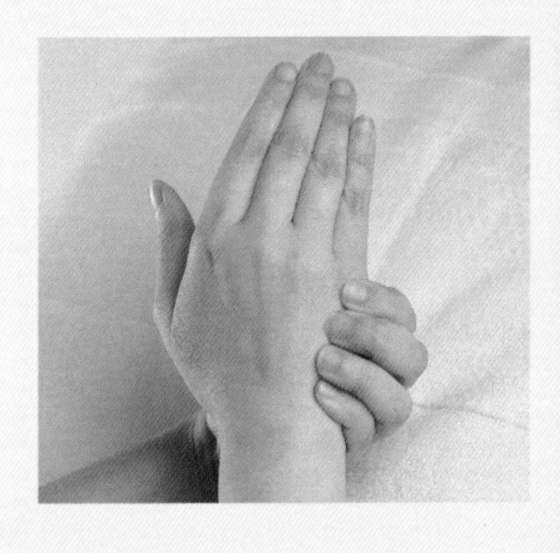

6 Spine

Walk your left thumb along the line indicated on your right hand.

7 Brain

Apply pressure with the left thumb directly to the top of your right thumb.

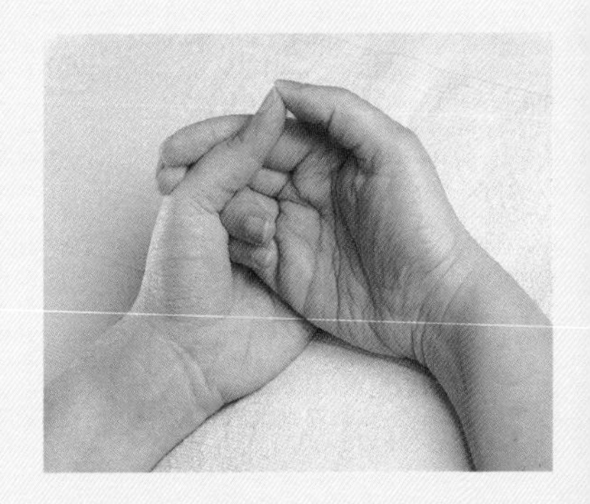

8

Shoulder/arm

Walk your left thumb over the area indicated on your right hand.

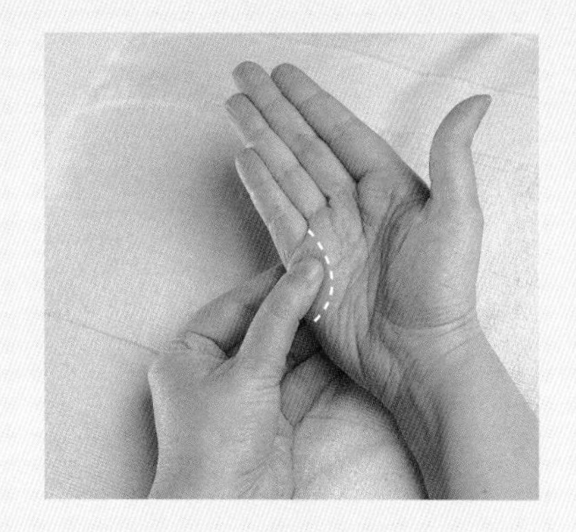

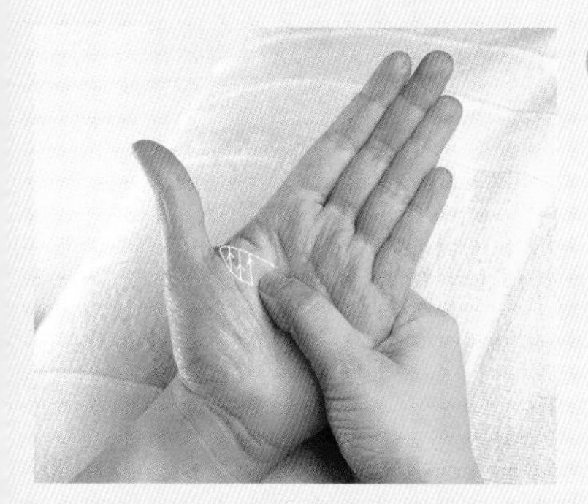

9

Stomach, pancreas and spleen

The reflex points for these organs are found on the left hand. Use your right thumb to walk the area indicated.

10

Colon

Walk your left thumb over the area of your right hand indicated.

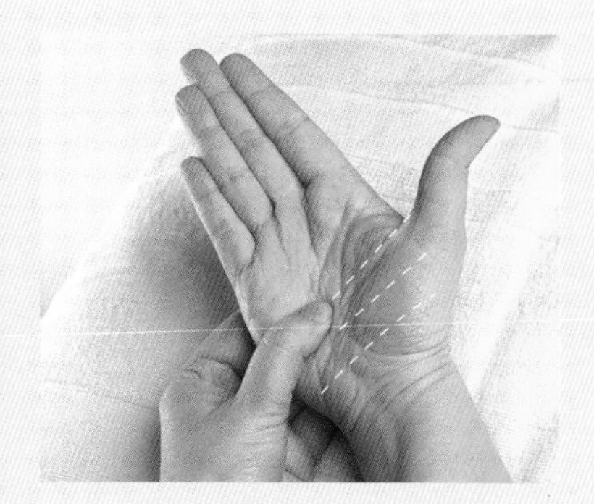

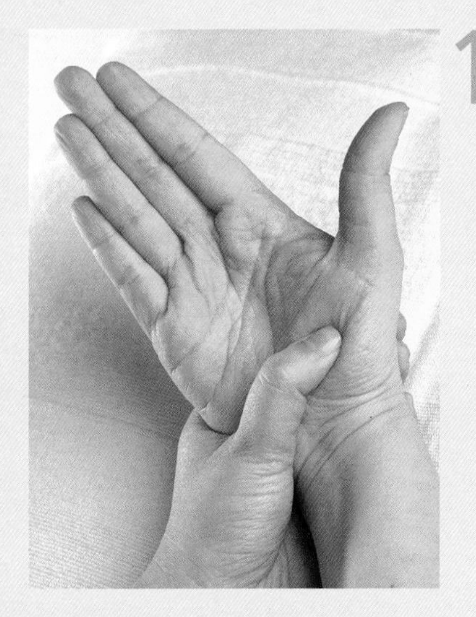

11 **Bladder**
Walk your left thumb over the fleshy pad just below the thumb of your right hand.

12 **Urethra**
Walk your left thumb from the bladder area towards the base of the index finger of your right hand.

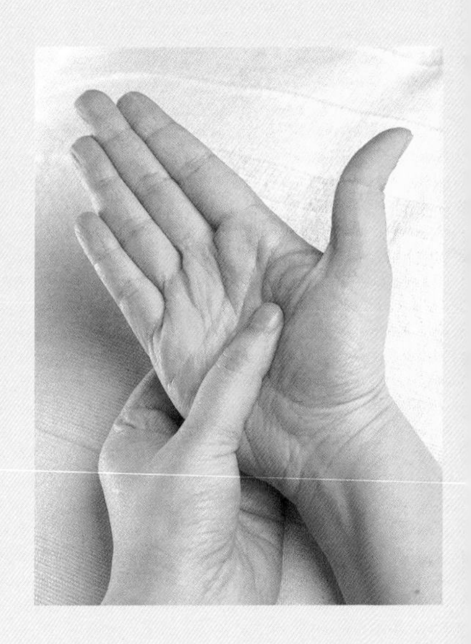

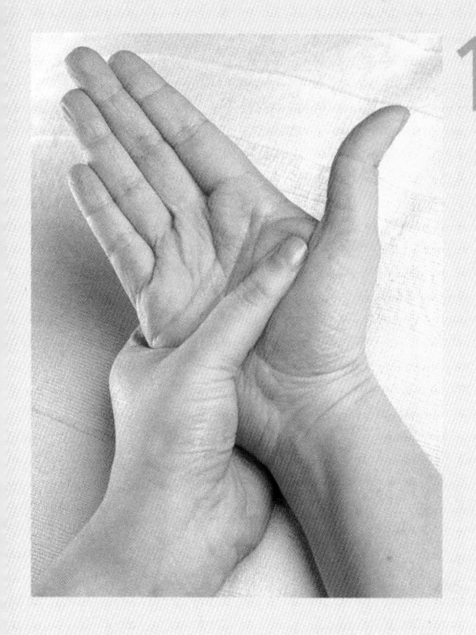

13

Kidneys

The reflex point for the kidneys is located where your thumb joins your hand. Exert pressure with the thumb of your left hand on your right hand.

14

Pelvic girdle (Uterus/prostate/ovaries/testes/Fallopian tubes/vas deferens)

Locate the reflex point just in front of your right wristbone. Use the third finger of your left hand to exert pressure on this area. Then use your index and middle fingers to work this area on both sides of your hand.

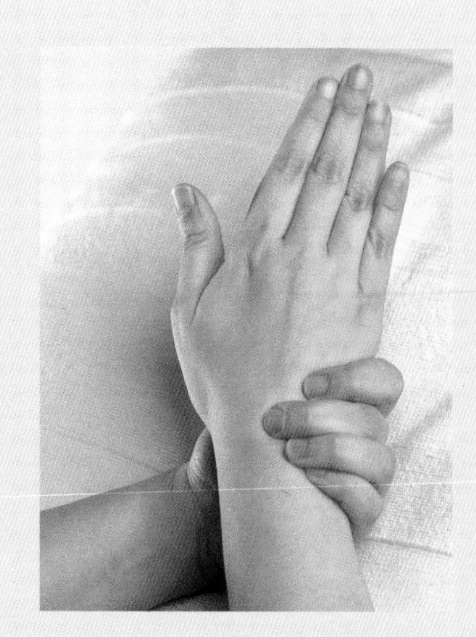

Reflexology *for* Health

Now you understand the principles of reflexology and have practised the techniques involved, you can use it to help family and friends feel relaxed and well. You can also use reflexology to help them through periods of ill-health. This section explains how to use reflexology effectively by evaluating the foot thoroughly and being aware of the areas of the foot associated with particular health problems. It also discusses stress and the role reflexology can play in its reduction.

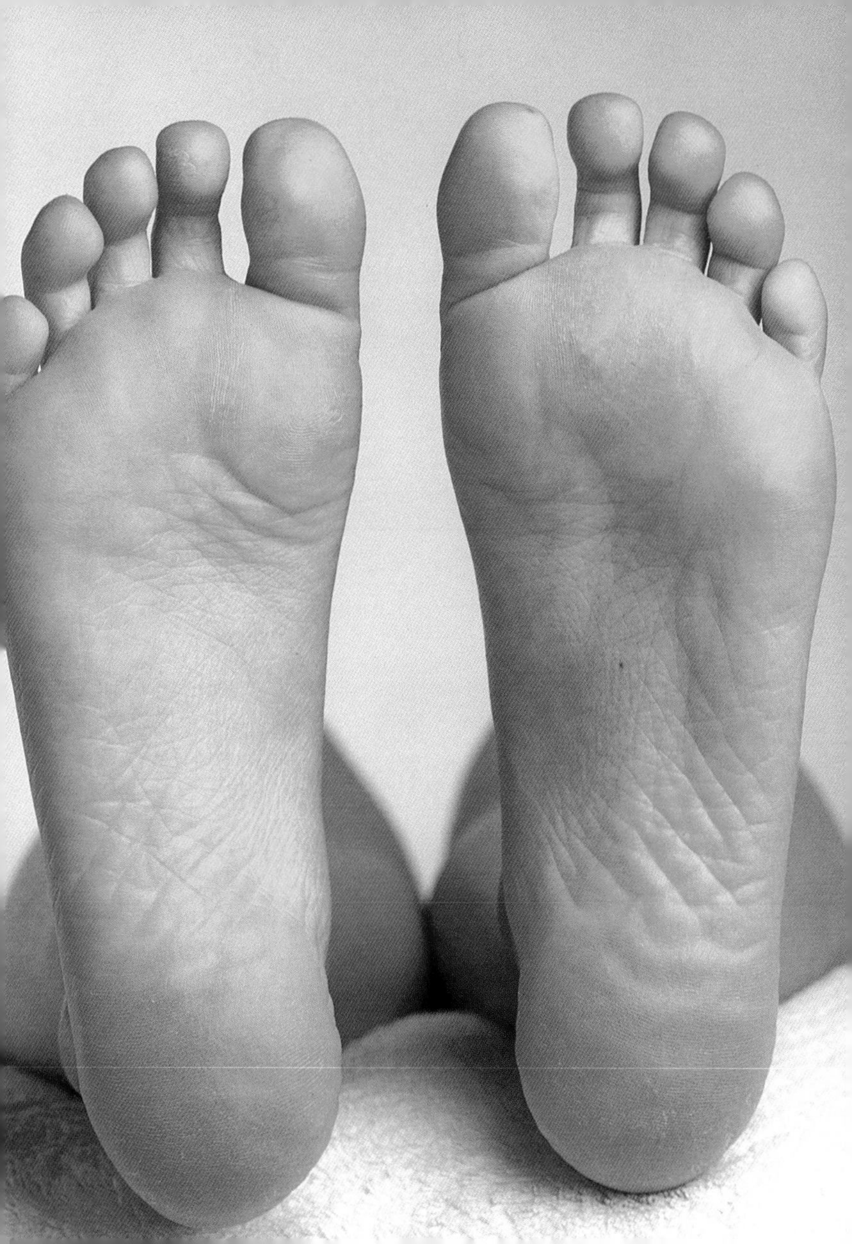

Don't diagnose!

When using reflexology, you should not try to diagnose what is wrong with the person you are treating. The beauty of reflexology is that, by careful observation of the foot and systematic treatment using the techniques and sequences already explained, you will be able to release tension throughout the body and help the body find its own equilibrium.

It is important, however, to learn how to evaluate the foot. From careful observation, you can begin to identify those zones of the body that are congested and therefore reflexes that might require some extra work. What you are looking for are areas of 'build-up' on the feet. These consist of deposits of calcium or lymph fluid which, according to reflexology theory, develop as a result of tension and stress. Some calcium deposits are hard (like, for example, those at the base of the toes), whereas others are soft and puffy. Corns and calluses are seen as external blockages that have developed in response to pressure, friction or repeated trauma. Build-up in any area will need to be worked on especially thoroughly.

Take a good look at your own feet and ask to examine the feet of friends. This way you will start to hone your observation skills and develop an ability to make a thorough evaluation.

If a friend tells you about a specific problem he or she is experiencing, you can refer to the chart on the following pages to identify those areas of the feet that might have build-up resulting from the problem. However, it is worth bearing in mind that symptoms can have many causes and you may not find any build-up in the area said to be associated with the symptoms described. If this is the case, press on and look carefully at the whole foot for areas of build-up that do need to be worked on.

Where to look on the foot when there is a problem

The chart that follows is a simple guide to those areas of the foot associated with some common health problems. It is not a diagnostic tool and is offered only as an aid to the detailed evaluation of the foot prior to a reflexology treatment.

Areas of foot associated with common health problems

Disorder	Area of Foot
Allergies	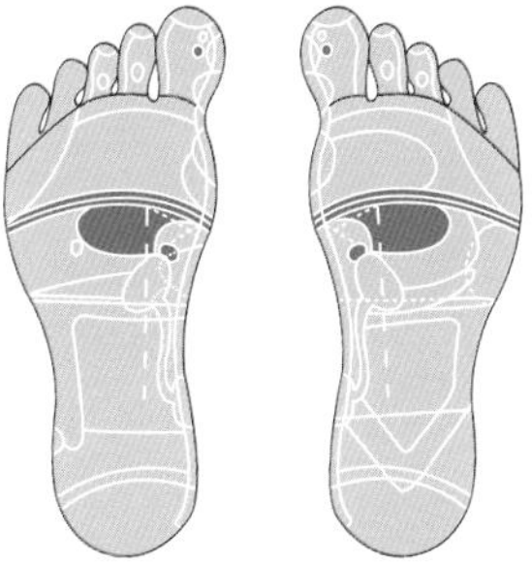
Anaemia	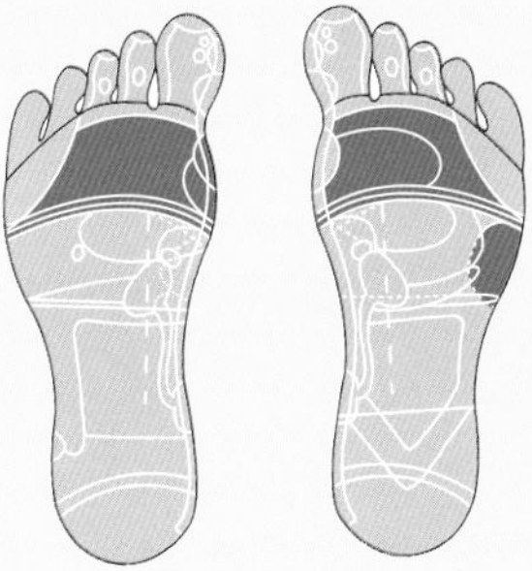
Asthma	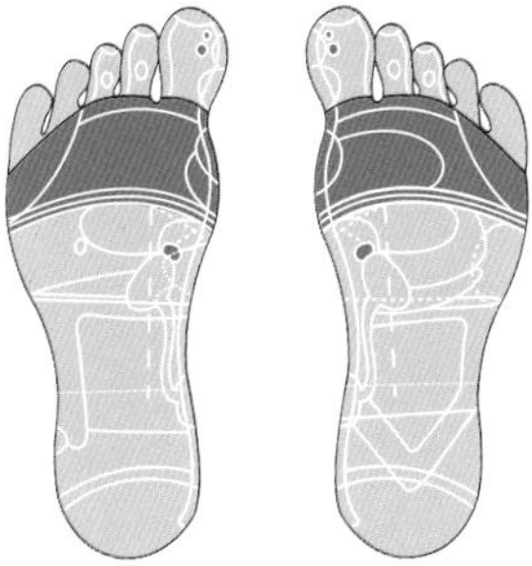

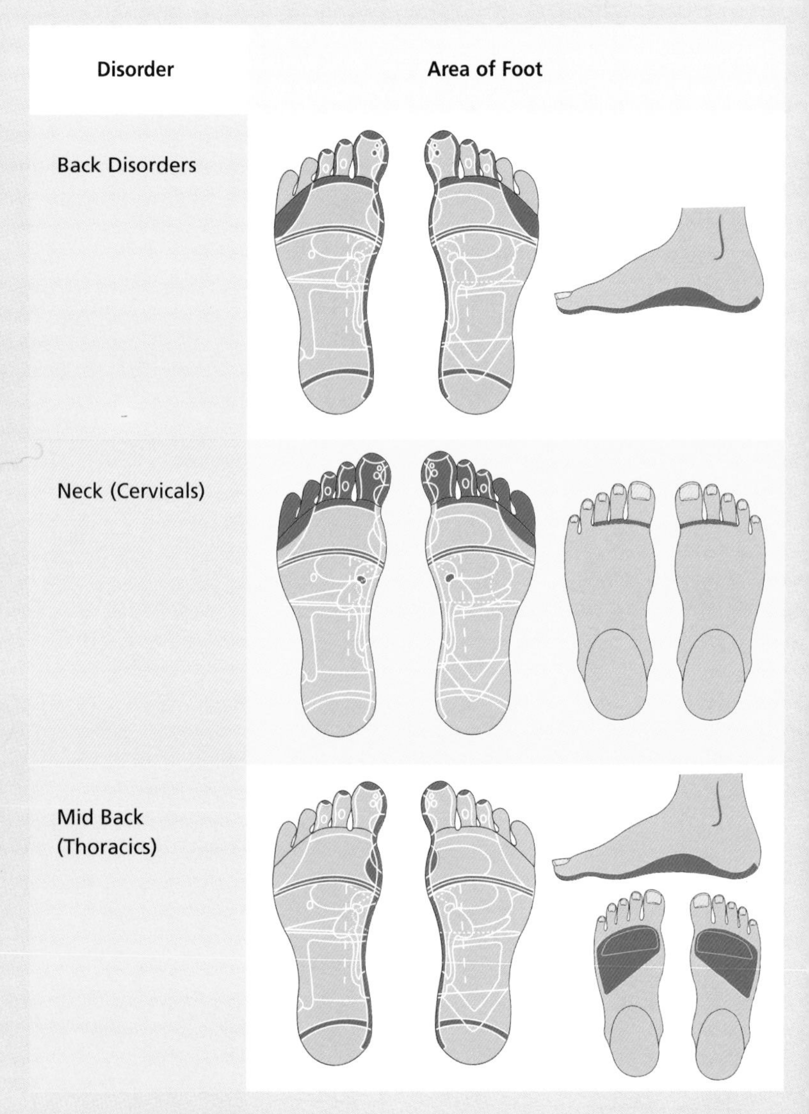
Disorder
Area of Foot
Back Disorders
Neck (Cervicals)
Mid Back
(Thoracics)

Disorder	Area of Foot
Lower back (Lumbars)	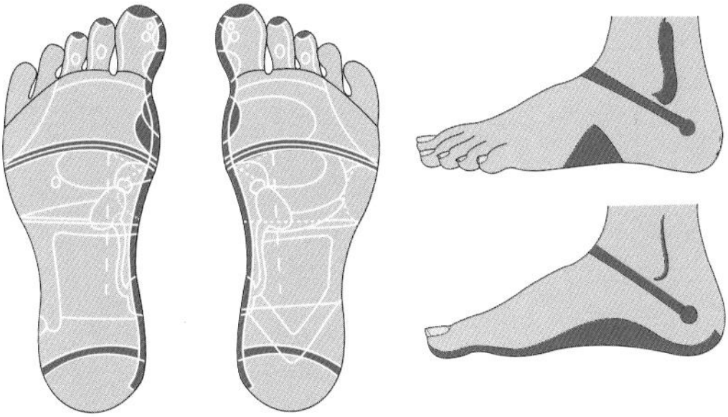
Lower back (Tailbone)	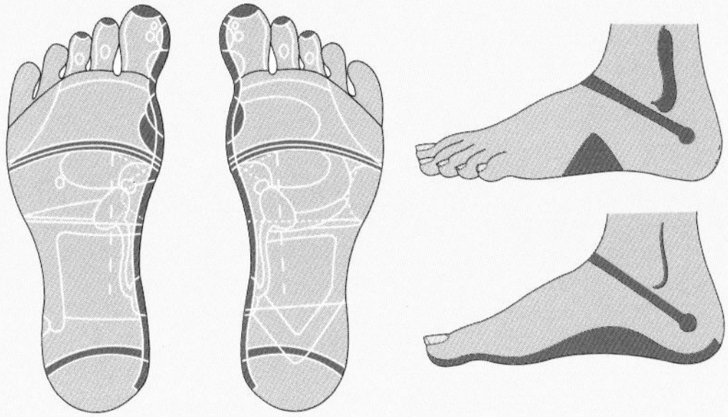
Bladder Disorders	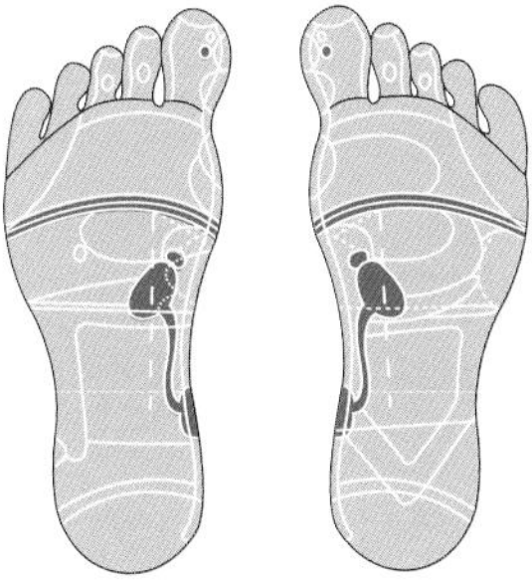

Disorder	Area of Foot
Constipation	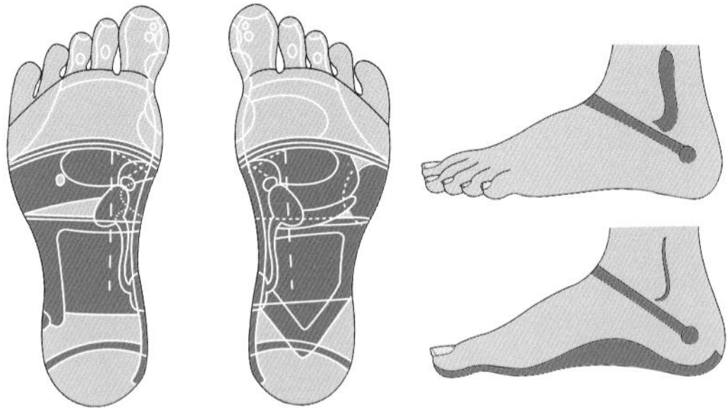
Depression	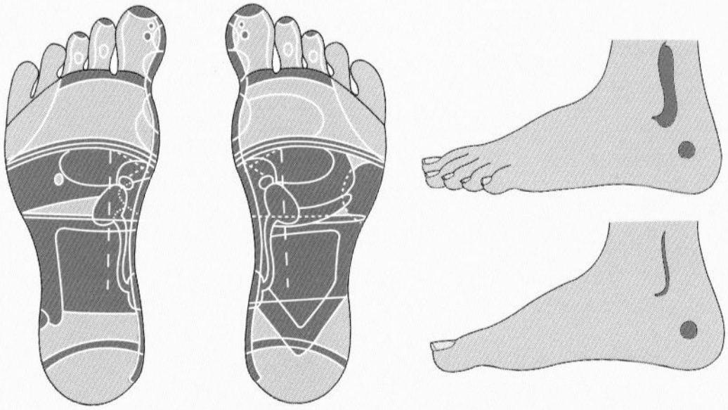
Dizziness (Vertigo)	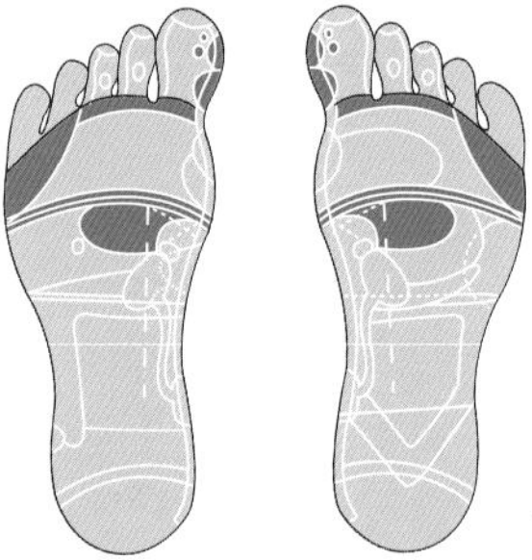

Disorder	Area of Foot
Earache	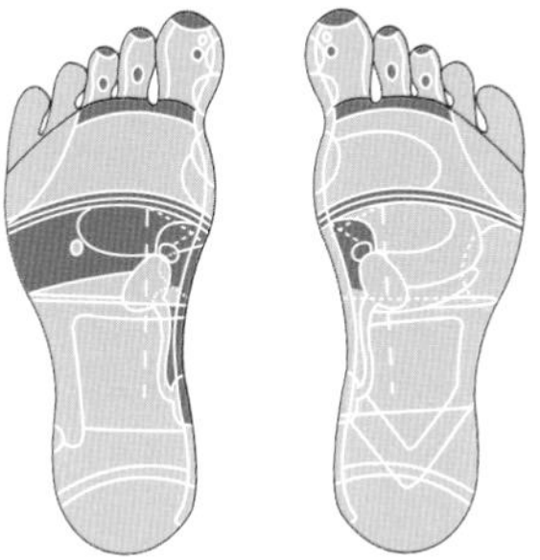
Eczema	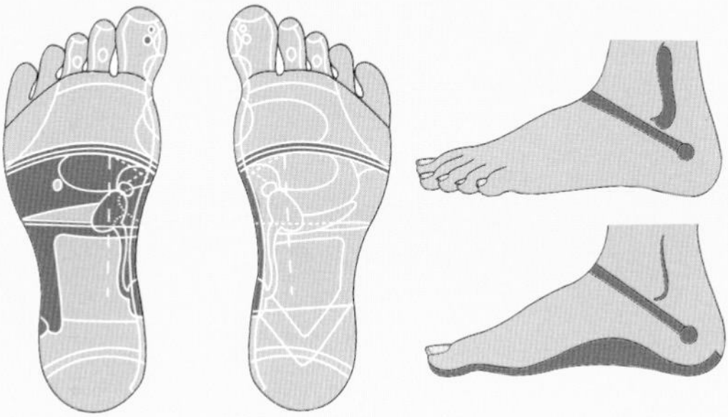
Female Disorders	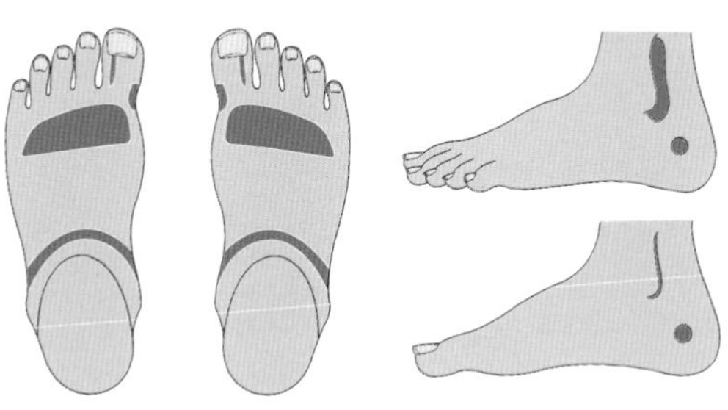

Disorder	Area of Foot
Flu	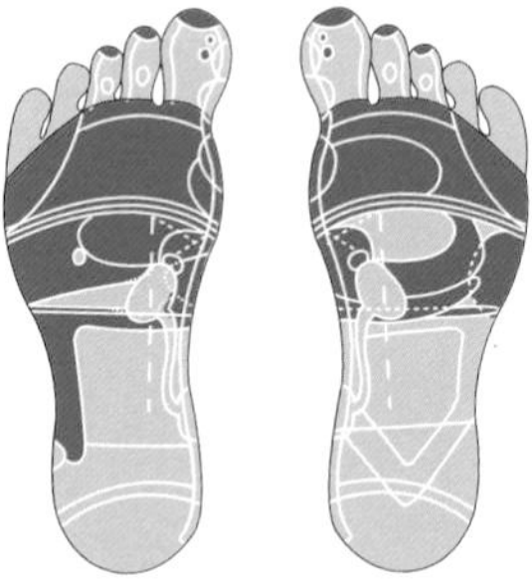
Flatulence	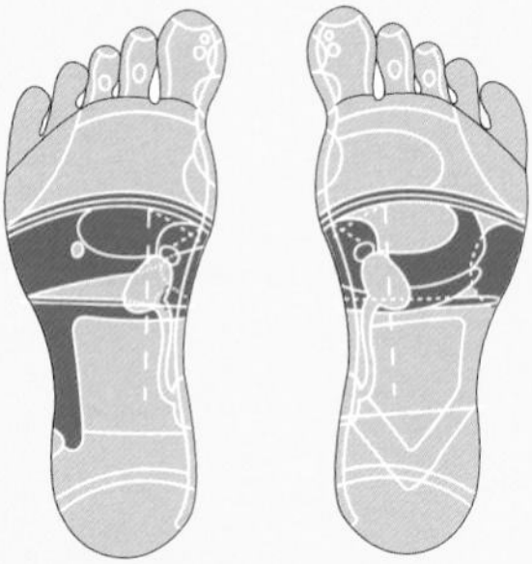
Headaches	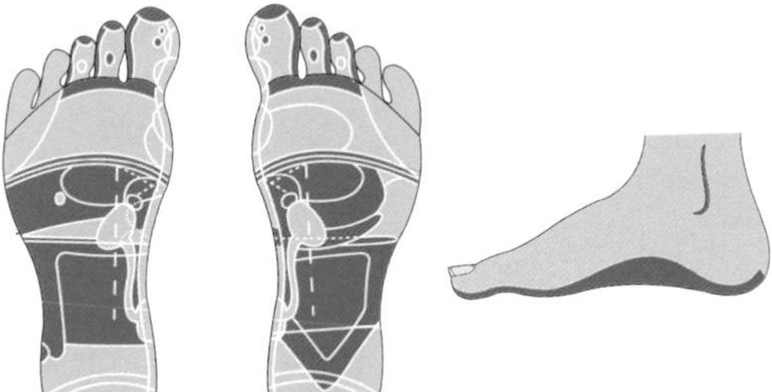

Disorder	Area of Foot
Haemorrhoids	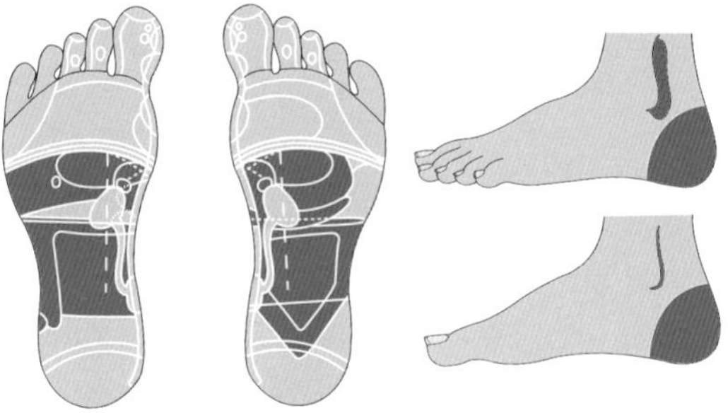
Shoulder Disorders	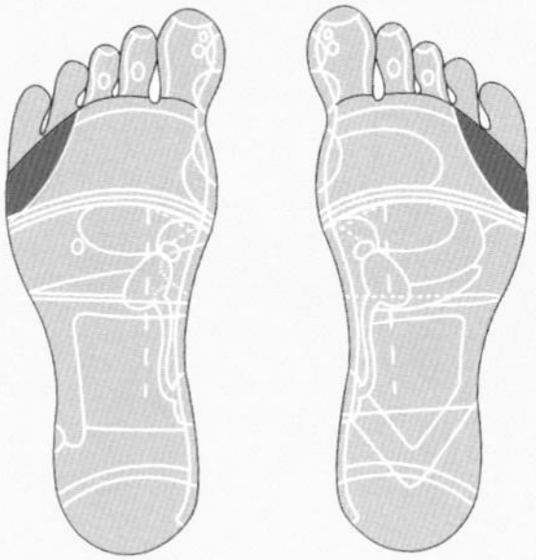
Sinusitis	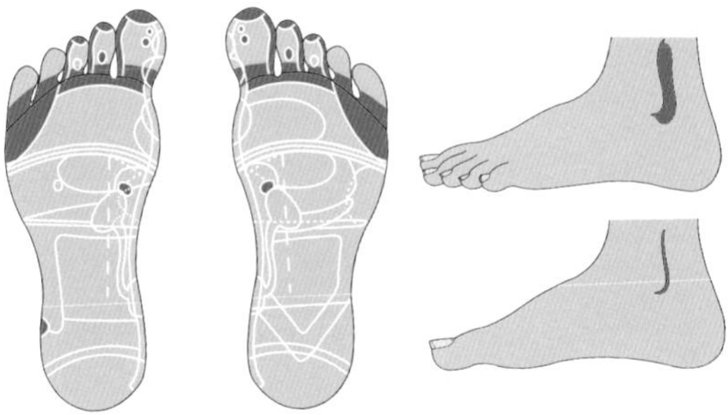

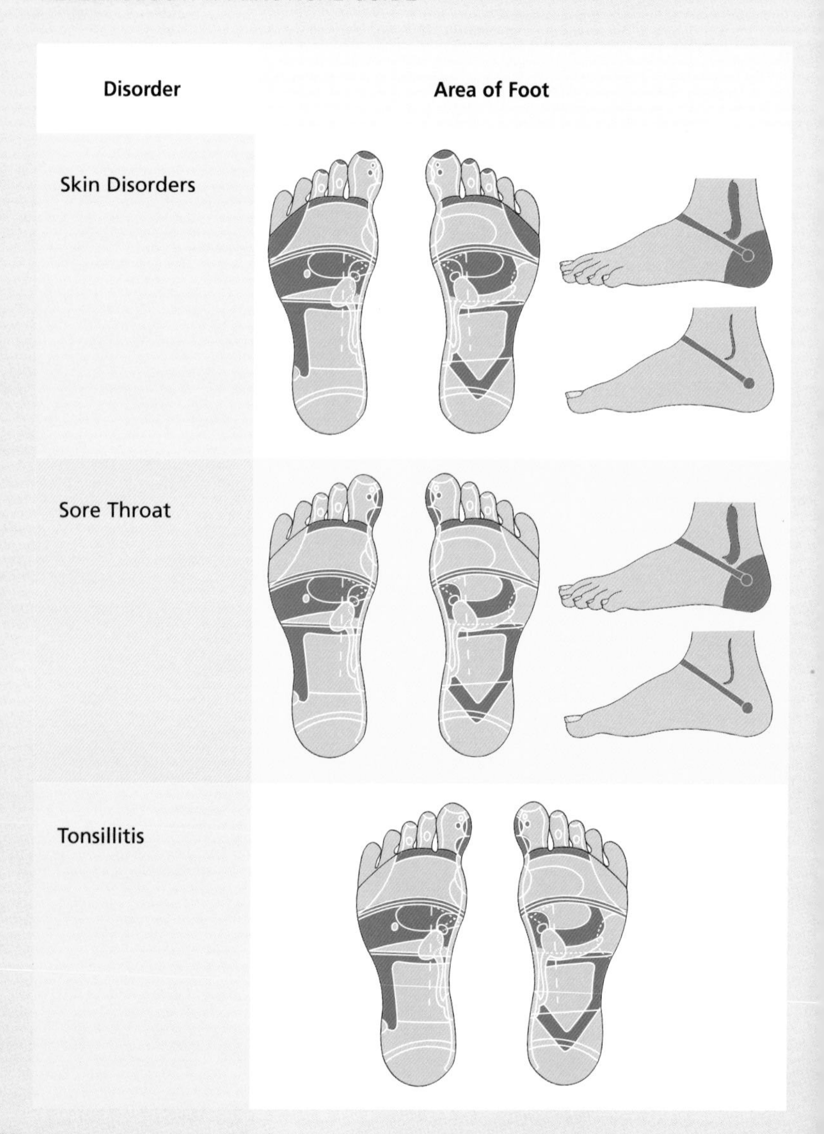

Disorder	Area of Foot
Skin Disorders	
Sore Throat	
Tonsillitis	

Tackling stress

There can be few people these days who do not, at times, suffer from too much stress; and the key to the success of reflexology is its ability to tackle adverse stress effectively.

What is stress?

Stress arises from our attitudes and reactions to events. If you think 'So what!' and really mean it, then you will experience no adverse stress, but this is usually easier said than done! Adverse stress steps in when we are unable to keep a sense of balance in a situation – whether it is travelling to work on a crowded train, finding enough money to pay the bills, or acrimonious arguments with friends or family. Of course, stress is not always negative. We all need a certain amount of it to perform at our optimum level and it's only when we are constantly stressed that it becomes harmful. And we now know that too much stress is linked to persistent ill-health and even to a lower life expectancy.

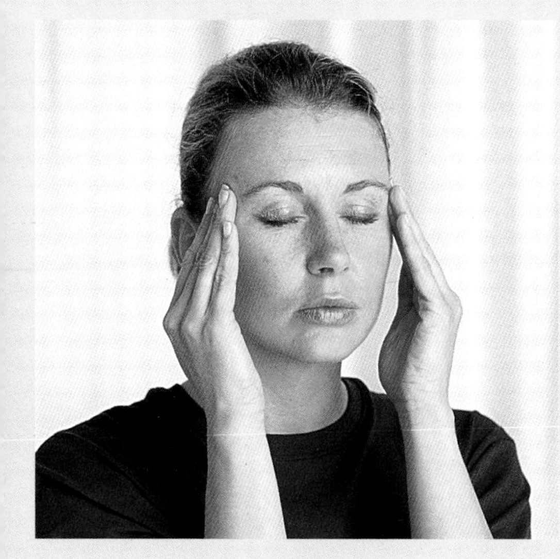

Many forms of massage can provide relief from stress, whether a simple massage of your forehead and temples with your fingertips, or a more thorough reflexology session.

The physiological link between illness and stress arises from our reaction to threats – something that comes from our evolutionary past as hunter-gatherers. We have a 'fight or flight' reaction to any perceived danger or risky situation: the levels of certain hormones, including adrenaline, dramatically increase, causing the heart beat to accelerate, blood pressure to rise and breathing to become more rapid. This is a natural and important reaction to danger that prepares us to respond appropriately. The buzz of a challenge at work or on the sports field can be positive and rewarding, but repeated provocation of these hormones, whether because we have too much work or because of other problems in our lives, exerts a huge strain on the cardiovascular and immune systems. Stress then becomes dangerous and can have a negative effect on health.

Managing stress

Regular reflexology treatments will, say therapists, reduce stress, improve health and increase that all-important sense of well-being.

Managing stress is vital if we are to stay well and live well. While regular reflexology treatments will help us to relax and even keep illness at bay, we should also look at other aspects of our lives that might need attention. It is important to eat healthily, take regular exercise, and ensure we get the sleep we need. We also need to look at the way we live our lives and consider whether changes in priorities, pace or direction might be beneficial.

Useful contacts

Association of Reflexologists
27 Old Gloucester Street
London WC1N 3XX
Tel: + 44 (0)870 5673320
www.aor.org.uk

Bayly School/British Reflexology Association
Monks Orchard
Whitbourne
Worcester WR6 5RB
Tel: +44 (0)1886 821207
E-mail (Bayly School):
bayly@britreflex.co.uk
E-mail (British Reflexology Association): bra@britreflex.co.uk
www.britreflex.co.uk

Holistic Association of Reflexologists
Holistic Healing Centre
92 Sheering Road
Old Harlow
Essex CM17 0JN
Tel: +44 (0)1279 429060
E-mail: ann@footreflexology.com
www.footreflexology.com

International School of Reflexology & Meridian Therapy
PO Box 68283
Bryanstan
2021
South Africa
Tel/Fax: +27 11 807 7184
www.vacuflex.com

International Federation of Reflexologists
76–78 Edridge Road
Croydon
Surrey CR0 1EF
Tel: +44 (0)20 8667 9458
E-mail: ifr44@aol.com
www.reflexology-ifr.com

Reflexologists' Society
PO Box 5422
Leicester LE2 2YG
Tel: +44 (0)870 6073241

Index